THE EXPRESSLANE DIET

A 21-Day Weight Loss Plan for People Who Enjoy Convenience, Fast and Frozen Foods

Audrey F. Blumenfeld, R.D., M.P.H.

toExcel

San Jose New York Lincoln Shanghai

The Expresslane Diet
A 21-Day Weight Loss Plan for People Who Enjoy Convenience,
Fast and Frozen Foods

This edition published by toExcel Press,
an imprint of iUniverse.com, Inc.

For information address:
iUniverse.com, Inc.
620 North 48th Street
Suite 201
Lincoln, NE 68504-3467
www.iuniverse.com

ISBN: 0-595-00004-5

Dedication

Dedicated with special thanks to my daughter, Rebecca
Ann Stern, and my beloved parents, Barbara and
Norman Blumenfeld, for their continued strength,
understanding and confidence, enabling me to fulfill
one more dream.

About the Author

Audrey F. Blumenfeld is a registered dietitian in private practice. She specializes in corporate fitness programs and nutrition counseling.

Having earned a Master's Degree from Columbia University, New York, Ms. Blumenfeld served as the Chief Clinical Dietitian for one of the Midwest's premiere medical centers, Michael Reese Hospital in Chicago. She is presently the national media spokesperson for Schering Plough Incorporated, a Fortune 500 Company. She also consults for physicians, hospitals, health centers and major corporations in the Midwest.

Table of Contents

Introduction

The evidence is in — and it's good news! Lots of convenience foods are nutritious and can help with weight control.

Manufacturers, supermarket managers and restaurants have become more sensitive to combining good nutrition with good taste. As a result, we can now buy a great variety of single-serving frozen, canned, processed and prepared convenience foods of premium quality. Breakfast, lunch and dinner entrees are all there on the shelves, to say nothing of the snacks for those of us who also enjoy "grazing."

In a special report from Tufts University (*Diet & Nutritional Letter*, volume 6, No. 1, March 1988), Dr. Jean Mayer recommends 99 frozen dinners and side dishes as "nutritionally sound." He evaluated the dinners on the basis of total fat, sodium, protein and palatability, as well as total calories. The trick of using these foods wisely lies in choosing others to use along with them that will round out your daily needs.

Dr. Michael Jacobson's "gloom ratings" in his book *The Fast Food Guide*, show us which fast foods to avoid. But it also shows us convenient fast foods that meet the nutritional criteria established by experts. It's all a matter of appropriate choice!

Biochemist and researcher Paul Saltman's *The California Nutrition Book* has also helped trash some of the popular diet myths about convenience foods. He says there isn't a good or bad food in and of itself. Saltman believes no food can be dismissed as "junk" and "there's no particular virtue in getting nutrients from natural foods." In fact, some candy bars and baked goods contain far more nutrients than apples or oranges. To be sure, they have more calories, but they also sometimes contain a greater percentage of nutrients to calories.

All this points to one thing: Our nutritional picture is often focused much too narrowly. It's time to evaluate foods on the basis of volume (amount eaten), balance (percentages of essential nutrients) and interactions with other foods and with our bodies. Saltman says instead of worrying what we will die from, Americans need to center in on how they can live better.

America's taste for fun, fast times, convenience, quality and variety continues to expand. About 45 percent of our nation's food dollar is spent on restaurant meals. At the same time, consumers are eager to learn which fast foods are nutritionally acceptable and to make healthy selections.

We are "pleasure seekers," and the kitchen is a low priority for many of us. Nearly 70 percent of women work outside the home, and many of them are single mothers. Few of us have time to cook, clean, work, pamper our mates, kids and pets, and still look like Mr. or Ms. Universe. Since food choices are simple in *The Expresslane Diet*, little time is spent in the kitchen. These meals almost make themselves.

I wrote *The Expresslane Diet* to accommodate no-time-to-spare lifestyles. I want to give Americans a quick, yet sound, weight loss plan — something they can follow, whether eating on the run, couching or cocooning in the privacy of their homes. And best of all, this approach doesn't involve spending an arm and a leg at a weight loss center or buying expensive, gimmicky foods or food supplements.

The Expresslane Diet offers more than most other food guides, calorie counters or brand-name nutritional references. It teaches you which convenience foods meet your body's nutritional needs for lower sodium, calories, fat and overall nutrient density and how to combine these foods appropriately. The 21-day plan has helped many folks lose up to seven pounds a week. Also, exchange lists of convenience foods and staples are included to help you plan your own menus and continue to lose weight. You need not be concerned about having to constantly tally calories or calculate food values. All the calculations have already been done. Your challenge is to select what most appeals to you from lists of recommended foods.

This is not a typical "diet" book. It is a way of life. It shows you how to incorporate nutritious quick-fix favorites while establishing new behaviors and learning maintenance tips that give you a permanent edge in the weight loss war.

All of the recommended convenience foods and menu plans meet the following nutritional criteria:

Main entrees contain no more than one-third of the maximum requirement for sodium.

Menus contain no more than 30 percent fat calories per day, and daily intake of cholesterol is less than 300 milligrams in keeping with the American Heart Association and the National Cancer Institute recommendations.

Daily menus contain a minimum of 45 grams of protein for women and 56 grams for men, which meets the U.S. Recommended Daily Allowance.

Emphasis is on complex carbohydrates and dietary fiber.

Daily menus do not exceed approximately 900 calories for women and 1,200 for men.

Participants need to take one all-purpose multiple vitamin with iron daily. The vitamin should not contain more than 100 percent of the U.S. RDA for any essential nutrients.

This is one rich food book that will leave dieters lighter on their feet.

CHAPTER 1

"Easy" Foods Can Be Good for You

America's new dinner, according to James Hightower, author of *Eat Your Heart Out*, is the "stuff of total food systems" owned, controlled and directed by Del Monte, General Mills, General Foods and other food giants. Hightower believes "cultural values" are being disregarded and dinner time is being converted to another "disposable product," manufactured uniformly and sold impersonally.

Is the fast food phenomenon dulling our senses? Does the unerring sameness of our convenience foods alter our perception of what food should be? Can we nutritionally "starve to death" from eating all that precooked, frozen, reheated, foil-and-plastic-packed food we get from vending machines, grocery store delis, gourmet and frozen food sections or fast-food pick-up stations?

The U.S. Senate Select Committee on Nutrition and Human Needs has expressed concern about this situation. Americans are becoming increasingly dependent on highly processed, packaged foods, resulting in a "mechanized approach to the provision of food." Over many years, such mechanization could pose nutritional as well as psychological problems. While the committee was primarily concerned with school and prison food services, the psychological impact of mechanized meals hits homes and restaurants as well.

We all derive pleasure from fine food that looks, smells and tastes good. However, other intangibles — feelings, perceptions and attitudes —are just as important as the food itself. That psychological gratification is deeply rooted and far more pervasive than a "home-made meal."

Fewer Cooks in the Kitchen

The decline of traditional cooking and home-made meals is far reaching. According to a survey by the Pillsbury Corporation through their publication, *What's Cookin?* the number of non-cooks eating on the run and the number of weight-conscious individuals increased dramatically between 1971 and 1986. Pillsbury refers to today's noncooks as the "Chase and Grabbits," describing them as young urbanites with two incomes, often single, childless and eating only out of necessity. Their typical fare consists of frozen convenience dinners, pizza and other carry-out, convenience-type foods. The Chase and Grabbits grew by as much as 136 percent, representing 26 percent of the 1986 sample, compared with only 11 percent of the 1971 sample. On the other hand, the number of "Happy Cookers" or those people taking personal satisfaction in cooking, decreased by 35 percent during this same time period — from 35 percent to only 15 percent. Similar decreases were seen in traditional cooking techniques. This study suggests while we want to eat right, we also want convenience. Clearly, convenience foods can be nutritious, too! For some nutrition-conscious individuals, this has meant eating more ready-made fish and chicken dishes, switching from whole milk to skim milk and eating more fresh or frozen fruits, vegetables and whole grains.

Competition in convenience foods abounds. Low-calorie options are especially plentiful. In fact, our society's concept of dieting and convenience are quite similar. We seek quick-fix results from diets without having to make major decisions or work hard. We want a plentiful array of quick-fix, convenient, portable, ready-made, heat-and-eat meals in minutes.

In the food arena, today's nutrition-conscious shopper has many options. Over the last several years, the influx of new, specialty, convenience-type products has been tremendous, primarily because we keep buying. Now shoppers can pick up everything from flowers and china to gourmet meals. How much more convenient could it be?

Diet carry-out service is even available in some parts of the country. For about $70 to $80 per week per person, customers are provided door-to-door delivery or convenient pick up. And best of all, menus can be tailored for weight loss or special situations, such as diabetic, low-cholesterol or low-sodium diets.

However, these local carry-out operations, while fundamentally sound, stand little chance competing against major food corporations with their product development, marketing, advertising and financial capacities. Still, as a famous songwriter once put it, "the times, they are a changing."

Have consumers entrusted big businesses to "leave dinner to them" because Americans don't know how to produce, process or prepare food anymore? Is Ms. Sally Simpleton relying on "Hamburger Helper" to get her through the week because she has forgotten or never knew how to prepare a meal that isn't pre-measured, preseasoned and sitting right there on the shelf?

I understand why women, in particular, take advantage of convenience foods. Most of us work and have youngsters, hectic schedules and competing demands to juggle. With more adults in the work force and individuals working longer hours, there is less free time to plan or prepare meals as we would like. In fact, food industry analysts tell us saving time ranks uppermost with most of us today. In 1986, the Food Marketing Institute showed that consumers were even more interested in saving shopping time than they had been just one year earlier. It appears we only shop for needed items and buy in bulk to avoid frequent trips to the grocery store.

"Convenience," "quick," "speedy" and "easy" have become the operative buzz words for today's cooks. Savvy cooks have learned to combine high-quality convenience items with staple ingredients from the cupboard, refrigerator or freezer. Why not use what little free time there is to foster knowledge in other areas besides cooking? Physical fitness, hobbies or merely enjoying quality time with our families and friends often outranks kitchen chores. We all have choices to make. Unfortunately, sometimes all we have after slaving over a hot stove is dishpan hands, a full stomach and perhaps memorable conversation.

Don't misunderstand. We're not breeding a society that objects to home cooking. Our lifestyles simply are not conducive to preparing elaborate meals. According to Louis Harris's *Inside America*, there emerges a nation in which four out of every ten adults neither have the patience, time or desire to prepare a "home-cooked meal." On any given day, one in three American adults eats at least one meal out. Between 10 and 12 percent buy take-out food on any given day.

According to recent reports from the National Restaurant Association, in 1993 the average consumer spent 43.0 percent of their food dollars on food eaten away from home. The average American (eight years old and older) eats out almost four times a week or approximately 198 times each year. Lunch is the meal eaten out most frequently, followed by dinner and breakfast least often. Men still dine out more frequently than women.

Restaurants and other food establishments have capitalized on information showing we eat on the run. More than half the American population, roughly 133 million people, eat out or buy to-go foods every single day. Nearly 33% of people eating out choose fast food. American cooking remains the choice cuisine, holding a 55% preference margin, with Italian next at 14%, Chinese at 12%, Mexican at 8%, French 2% and Japanese 2%.

Today, single-person households and two-worker families are the sociological forces that continue to feed our desire to eat out. While people differ in their individual food preferences, when grouped according to family, age and lifestyle, most share a common desire for quality food. Convenience dining has become a "way of life" for almost all Americans — regardless of age, sex or race — because it meets our needs for quality, taste and ease of preparation.

We all like to spend a leisurely evening at home enjoying a wonderful meal. Since we prefer to be home at night, Americans tend to eat out at noon. Even when we do eat at home, we seldom cook everything from scratch. Preparing a meal takes time for planning, shopping, cooking, serving and cleaning up. That's a big chunk from the estimated two and a half hours of free time most of us have each day. Then, too, everyone wants and needs a "break."

Even though costs for dining out have gone up faster than costs for food we can make at home, there's that intangible value on our time that influences us. When was the last time you cuddled up on the sofa or read or spent time with others after work without thinking about preparing supper or cleaning up afterwards? Can you give your toddler an unhurried bubble bath — or do you have to get dinner on the table? What about spending an evening with a friend playing cards, tennis or taking dance lessons? Just plain relaxing in front of the TV might also be a welcome change of pace.

The One-Handed Society

Some people think of convenience foods as "finger foods," "no-think foods," "easy to grab" or "commuter foods" that usually require no utensils, don't drip, spill, crumble or require inordinate attention other than hand-to-mouth coordination. But today's quick bites are more than convenient. Many are portion controlled, available in single servings, composed of quality ingredients and geared for rapid consumption.

Finger foods are the ultimate convenience foods, fitting our casual lifestyles. They're easy to buy and prepare when we have "more important" things to worry about. They are our "no dinner dinner" and can be exotic or plain. Half the fun is how they're presented. When served with style and panache, a "snack" can be a jazzy meal. We can enjoy finger foods at our desks, walking, biking, flying or just relaxing at home.

Have you noticed the new "one-handed society" of grazers? Because of the nature of our jobs or our need or desire to exercise, some of us are forced to eat on the run. We aren't "clocked" into specified meal times. If we want to eat lunch at three in the afternoon, it's no problem to pick up something or pop a quick-fix meal into the microwave. (Interestingly, about 60 percent of Americans have access to microwaves at work.) Some supermarkets and restaurants are open 24 hours a day. And don't forget the drive-through fast-food possibilities.

So what's happening to meet this "convenience" trend? Manufacturers and marketers alike have responded to our desire for sophistication coupled with our concern for health and wellness. Food developers continue to offer uncounted light, luscious and fun foods — many reflecting a trend toward healthier eating. Lighter meats, poultry and fish, combination vegetable dishes, pasta and potato creations tempt us from freezer shelves. Many of these foods have been prepared with less fat, fewer calories and less sodium than regular versions.

"Convenience" has not limited our food choices, either. Diet-conscious patrons can select lighter fare, including sandwiches, pizza, soups, salads or appetizers. Entrees, meal accompaniments of fruit, vegetables and assortments of grain foods also are available. Best of all, there are desserts you need not desert, provided they are accounted for in your total daily intake. Remember, prudent food patterns don't have to exclude an element of fun!

Also, by using food guides and labels along with this diet's brand-name recommendations, you can judge products on the basis of comparable nutritional values of similar foods.

Check Those Labels

Frozen foods and convenience products usually have labels that can guide you to nutritious choices. The labels give us calories, protein, carbohydrate, fat, sodium and cholesterol content. The percentage of the U.S. RDA for protein, vitamins A and C, as well as calcium and iron should be considered.

Calories, fat, cholesterol and sodium are important for weight control. Experts advise limiting fat to no more than 30 percent of the total daily calories. To translate grams of fat on labels into serving sizes, simply visualize that for every 5 grams of fat, you have the equivalent of one level teaspoon of fat such as butter, margarine, salad oil, etc. Fats contribute about two and one-quarter times the calories per gram as proteins or carbohydrates. By merely cutting back on fat, you can save a bundle of calories.

Current recommendations limit sodium to 2,400 milligrams per day. Therefore, it makes good sense to buy entrees that are moderately low in sodium. Since all other food accompaniments — rolls, margarine, salad dressing, etc. — also contain sodium, it's easy to get too much without realizing it. With care, though, you can restrict fat, calories and salt — and lose weight. Start by reading labels.

As you learn and understand more, your tastes will change accordingly. You don't have to compromise! That's why Dave Jennings, vice-president of sales at Stouffer's Foods, feels his company has achieved long-standing success throughout time. Stouffer's offers gourmet quality products that match American's needs for lighter meals with their line of Lean Cuisine entrees. And while quality has a price, consumers appear willing to pay for it— as long as it meets their needs and something doesn't come along that's just as good but less expensive.

Despite the fact that some consumer's view supermarkets as storehouses for thousands of items, there are far fewer nutritional choices than one might imagine. Many of the old established brand-name products have been corralled by consumer product companies. Let's face it. We all have favorite brand-name manufacturers — LaChoy for Chinese, Ortega for Mexican, Dannon for yogurts and Jay's, Lay's and Nabisco for chips or snacks. The Del Monte Corporation has led the fruit pack for years, with crafty ads telling us they have been with us throughout our lives — "from womb to tomb."

Regardless of who has satisfied our cravings for food, Americans are making great strides to change long-standing unhealthy food patterns. At the same time, we face a time crunch. Longing for quality food, convenience and fun, we are opting for "healthier" convenience products and fast-food dining.

Fast Food Can Fit

Fast food operations are definitely changing to try to accommodate fast times and health trends. Menus are lighter, more nutritious and tastier. Burgers have come a long way, baby! If we had only stayed with the fifteen cent plain hamburger of the 1950s, our nutritional status wouldn't have been compromised. It's the gooey cheese laced between layers of refined bread topped with mayonnaise, salad dressing, pickle chips, bacon strips and sauteed vegetables that stimulated the salivary glands. Guts, butts and waistlines will not expand if we opt for carefully selected items from salad and baked potato bars, cafeteria-style top-your-own sandwich areas featuring lean roast beef, baked or broiled chicken or fish and hearty vegetable stocks. For desserts we can choose fresh fruit, ice milk or yogurt instead of the standard malts, shakes or sundaes.

Restaurants have changed in other ways. They now provide subtle lighting, more privacy, natural earthy atmospheres for comfortable home-like seating, as well as marble, mirrors, brass and glass for the sophisticated appetites. Moreover, restaurants often offer parents more time alone, providing jungle gyms, merry-go-rounds, puzzles, coloring books and games galore to pacify children. Many of us gain our first exposures to fast food spots because our kids want to go there. Undoubtedly we have advertisers to thank for that.

How big is this fast food market? To date, there are more than 55,000 fast food restaurants competing for the American greenback. In 1985, according to the trade journal *Restaurants and Institutions*, fast food sales accounted for more than $43 million. The U.S. Department of Agriculture (USDA) stated that fast food sales jumped by 40 percent between 1977 and 1985. Today, the USDA states that almost five out of every 10 dollars exchanged over a restaurant counter occurs in a fast-food spot. In fact, in the 1980s the average amount of money an American spent on fast foods was $200 per year, with increases certain in the future. The top five fast-food chains drawing one-half of all profits include McDonald's, Burger King, Kentucky Fried Chicken, Wendy's and Hardee's. Amazingly, one McDonald's restaurant is built every 15 hours somewhere around the world, with total corporate sales topping $11 billion per year. Don't you think that these chains must be offering more than "a good time for the great taste" or "food for fast times"?

Americans have changed. We won't fight convenience. Instead, we'll move ahead — strengthen our nutritional knowledge and work to redefine dietary myths on convenience dining.

After reading *The Expresslane Diet*, you'll see there is indeed a place for convenience food in our prudent plans without depersonalizing dinner or the diner. Let me show you how you can enjoy the best of all food worlds by complimenting and combining fresh, convenience, prepared, fast and frozen foods while safely losing weight and having a great time doing it. *The Expresslane Diet* is the answer!

CHAPTER 2

The Plan

Calories aren't the most important part of dieting. While they count, the components of the diet — proteins, carbohydrates, fat, sodium and fiber — determine nutritional value. Menu plans, calorie counting and calculations for daily percentages of carbohydrate, protein, fat, cholesterol, sodium and dietary fiber have already been done for you in *The Expresslane Diet*. Also, a supplementary exchange system incorporating ten different food groups gives you the freedom to plan your own menus, using fresh, frozen, ready-prepared and fast foods.

Menus from *The Expresslane Diet* provide the best examples of healthy ways to combine convenience, combination dishes, fruits, vegetables, whole-grain breads and low-calorie desserts. This book balances the U.S. RDAs for adults, yet provides variety, taste and appeal without excessive calories, sodium, fat, cholesterol or sugar. Most importantly, *The Expresslane Diet* includes foods Americans have avoided over the last few years, such as lean red meats and low-fat dairy products. This balanced approach reduces the risk of a diet deficient in folic acid, iron, zinc, vitamin B6, magnesium and calcium.

While breakfast, lunch and dinner menus in *The Expresslane Diet* can't be mixed and matched, you can change the order of the 21 daily menus. It's the daily total that counts — not one meal or a couple of isolated figures.

The Expresslane Diet provides two separate diet plans: a 21-day 900-calorie plan for women and a 1,200-calorie plan for men. Each day's plan contains about 60 percent of calories from carbohydrates, with emphasis on high-fiber complex carbohydrates. These are whole-grain breads, cereals, fruits and vegetables. Approximately 20 percent of calories are from protein, with a minimum of 45 and 55 grams for women and men, respectively. Only 22 percent of calories are from fat, with polyunsaturated and monounsaturated fats being used instead of saturated. Cholesterol is limited to 150 milligrams and sodium averages

2,200 milligrams per day. This program conforms to the American Heart Association's "Healthy Heart" guidelines, as well as standards set by the National Cancer Institute. These require 30 percent or less fat, moderately low sodium, low-cholesterol and overall low calories.

You can anticipate losses — up to as much as seven pounds a week — until you reach your desired or ideal body weight range. You can opt to repeat the 21-day *Expresslane Diet* cycle for as many times as it takes you to reach your desired weight. Or you can plan your own menus using *The Expresslane Diet* Exchange System. However, *The Expresslane Diet* should be followed for the full 21-days before repeating any day's menus or using the exchange system. Both systems are designed with separate minimum/maximum maintenance guidelines for continued weight control.

The Expresslane Diet paves the way to enjoying quick, tasty and nutritious foods while attaining and maintaining a trimmer you.

To determine your desired body weight, use the following height and weight table designed by the Metropolitan Life Insurance Company. These weights are based on low mortality for ages 25 to 59 years. Weights are adjusted for frame size. Adjustments include five pounds of clothing for men and three pounds for women. Height includes shoes with one-inch heels.

METROPOLITAN HEIGHT AND WEIGHT TABLE

Height (ft,In)	Men Small Frame	Medium Frame	Large Frame	Women Small Frame	Medium Frame	Large Frame
4'10"				102-111	109-121	118-131
4'11"				103-113	111-123	120-134
5'0"				104-115	113-126	122-137
5'1"				106-118	115-129	125-140
5'2"	128-134	131-141	138-150	108-121	118-132	128-143
5'3"	130-136	133-143	140-153	111-124	121-135	131-147
5'4"	132-138	135-145	142-156	114-127	124-138	134-151
5'5"	134-140	137-148	144-160	117-130	127-141	137-155
5'6"	136-142	139-151	146-164	120-133	130-144	140-159
5'7"	138-145	142-154	149-168	123-136	133-147	143-163
5'8"	140-148	145-157	152-172	126-139	136-150	146-167
5'9"	142-151	148-160	155-176	129-142	139-153	149-170
5'10"	144-154	151-163	158-180	132-145	142-156	152-173
5'11"	146-157	154-166	161-184	135-148	145-159	155-176
6'0"	149-160	157-170	164-188	138-151	148-162	158-179
6'1"	152-164	160-174	168-192			
6'2"	155-168	164-178	172-197			
6'3"	158-172	167-182	176-202			
6'4"	162-176	171-187	181-207			

Weights at ages 25-59 based on lowest mortality. Weight in pounds according to frame (in indoor clothing weighing 5 lbs. for men, 3 lbs. for women: height in shoes with 1-in. heels).

Source: 1983 Metropolitan Height and Weight Tables, Metropolitan Life Insurance Company.

Before beginning *The Expresslane Diet* Program, it's important to review the following guidelines.

Guidelines

- Before beginning any weight loss program, it's always smart to visit your physician. Tell him or her what you plan to do and ask about any restrictions. Inform family members what the diet is and how it works in order to enforce self-esteem. During the program you may also want to consult with your physician to advise of your progress.

- Tell someone important to you that you want to lose weight. Ask that person's help and support.

- Take a before and after picture of yourself. You'll want to see how quickly you change.

- Purchase an accurate bathroom scale. A digital is preferable since it gives a more specific reading. Weigh in once or twice a week at approximately the same time of day and preferably in your birthday suit.

- Purchase appropriate measuring utensils for weighing and measuring foods. A small food scale is an inexpensive but valuable investment. To gauge its accuracy, weigh out one stick of margarine. Your scale should register one-fourth of a pound or 4 ounces. Be sure to level amounts of fats or other foods measured in spoons. You'll be amazed how quickly you will be able to gauge portions!

- Since it's very difficult to get a proper balance of nutrients on less than 1,400 calories, you must take a daily multiple vitamin and mineral supplement. It should contain no more than 100 percent of RDAs. Women, in particular, should select a supplement containing vitamin B6, magnesium, calcium, iron and zinc nutrients that are often lacking in a woman's diet. Suggested brands include Centrum, Theragran M or One-A-Day Essential with Iron.

- Drink four to six 8-ounce glasses of water daily. Tea, coffee and low-sodium broth don't count in this total. If you find drinking water difficult, space it out. Try drinking half a glass each hour. For better taste add fresh lemon or lime juice and serve ice cold.

- Keep a daily food diary, detailing all foods and beverages consumed throughout the day. In addition, include the following circumstances under which you are eating:

- Time of day
- Place
- Disposition (how you're feeling)
- Who you're eating with
- What you're doing besides eating (watching TV, reading). This diary should be kept during the diet phase of this program and during maintenance. This is a great help for modifying certain food-related behaviors that threaten your success.

■ Don't skip meals. Don't go below 900 calories. You must eat all foods in the specified portions to ensure balanced nutrition.

■ With the exception of free fluids and permissible spices and herbs, you may not add any food, condiment or beverage to this diet. No alcohol is permitted.

■ To avoid forgetting what to eat, carry along a copy of this diet for ready reference. It's best to plan where, what and how much you're supposed to be eating before going out. Three separate weekly shopping lists have been provided to make getting ready easier.

■ Don't count calories! Calorie counting and calculations for carbohydrates, protein, fat, cholesterol, sodium and fiber have been done for you.

■ Follow *The Expresslane Diet* for the full 21-day cycle before repeating any day's menus or using the exchange system. You can opt to repeat the 21-day cycle for as many times as it takes you to reach your desired weight. If, after maintenance, you gain a few pounds, you can always restart the program.

■ Daily breakfasts, lunches and dinners are not interchangeable. You may, however, follow any daily menu order you wish. For example, you may prefer to begin with breakfast, lunch and dinner menus from day twenty-one and end with those from day one. You are also free to flip-flop any lunch or dinner menu of the same day if it's more convenient for you. It's the daily total that counts!

■ If you are unable to finish all of the permissible foods in any given day, don't add leftovers to the next day's food allowance.

■ Carefully check menu portions and serving sizes of all convenience-type products before purchasing them. Many are available in several different sizes. Remember, portion control remains paramount.

- If your local supermarket doesn't stock a specified product, don't hesitate to substitute a comparable convenience item. However, food values must closely approximate those used in *The Expresslane Diet*. Suggested guidelines are listed in the food substitution section.

- When a meal specifies one-half sandwich or entree, simply take the other half home or share it with a friend. Quit the "Clean Plate Club." It's better to "waste it than waist it!"

- Stock fruit, vegetable and whole-grain meal accompaniments in your school locker, backpack, briefcase or office refrigerator.

- If you go off the plan, don't penalize yourself or become unduly discouraged. Don't wait to start it again next week. Get right back on track with your next meal. You are only human. Be patient, and don't expect perfection from yourself.

- Reward yourself with non food items for every 10-pound drop in weight. Rewards might include a new hair style, a facial or massage, theatre tickets, a new outfit or a special piece of sports equipment for your new image.

- Monitor your weight loss creatively. Try charting losses on a bar graph. Remember to compete with yourself only! Give yourself credit for appropriate food choices and always keep yourself challenged. You'll be better equipped to control your eating and consequently your weight.

- Exercise for at least 30 minutes three times a week. Take an active role in reshaping your lifestyle by finding an activity you enjoy. Experiment until you find a workout setting and activities that keep you stimulated and interested. Remember, there is no right way to live! Different strokes for different folks.

- For oral gratification, you're free to chew up to one package of sugar-free gum daily. No other dietetic or diabetic candies, cookies or cakes should be used.

- Any noncaloric sweetener, such as saccharin, aspartame or acesulfame-K, may be used in moderation to flavor cereal, beverages and fruits. Acceptable sweeteners are marketed under the banner of Equal, Nutrasweet, Sweet 'n Low or Sweet One. Avoid sweeteners containing fructose, mannitol and sorbitol. These are sugars and do contain calories.

■ Unless directed by a physician, don't take any laxatives or diuretics (water pills). Laxatives should not be necessary as you will be eating a moderate supply of dietary fiber. Remember you can jeopardize stores of valuable electrolytes — sodium and potassium in particular — if you abuse these medications. And retaining water shouldn't be a problem since this plan is moderately low in dietary sodium.

THE EXPRESSLANE DIET
CUMULATIVE NUTRITIONAL ANALYSIS
(21 DAYS)

WOMEN'S DIET PROGRAM

Carbohydrate (grams) 131
Protein (grams) 46
Fat (grams) 22
Cholesterol (milligrams) 138
Calories 907
Sodium (milligrams) 1,995

Percent of Total Calories
Carbohydrate 58%
Protein 20%
Fat 22%

MEN'S DIET PROGRAM

Carbohydrate (grams) 179
Protein (grams) 59
Fat (grams) 29
Cholesterol (milligrams) 159
Calories 1,216
Sodium (milligrams) 2,319

Percent of Total Calories
Carbohydrate 59%
Protein 19%
Fat 22%

FREE BEVERAGES FOR
THE EXPRESSLANE DIET

- Coffee — regular or decaffeinated, hot or iced without added sugar

- Tea — regular or decaffeinated, hot or iced without added sugar

- Club Soda or Carbonated Water without added sugar

- Mineral Water or Regular Tap Water

- Sugar-Free Tonic

- Sugar-Free Soda (any flavor) with no more than 1 gram of carbohydrate per 6 fluid ounce serving

- Sugar-Free Fruit Flavored Drinks (any flavor) with no more than 4 calories per serving

- Juice from one fresh lemon or lime to flavor water or soda

The following 21 daily menus are designed for women from the ages of 22 to 59 years.

WOMEN   DAY 1

BREAKFAST:

4 "Bite Size" Sunsweet Pitted Prunes
1 1/2 Hungry Jack Extra Rich Buttermilk Biscuits
2 teaspoons Smucker's Fruit Spread (any flavor)
Coffee or Tea with sugar substitute

LUNCH:

"Stuffed Baked Potato"
    1 medium Plain Baked Potato topped with:
        1/2 cup raw Broccoli pieces
        1/2 cup raw sliced Mushrooms
        1 tablespoon minced raw Onion
        1/4 cup Lite-Line Low-Fat Cottage Cheese
        1/2 small Tomato, diced
        1 tablespoon Kraft Bacon & Tomato Reduced-Calorie
            Salad Dressing
Coffee, Tea or "Free Beverage"

DINNER:

1 (10 ounce) Frozen Banquet Green Pepper Steak entree
1 cup plain baked Acorn, Butternut or Hubbard Squash topped
with:
    1 teaspoon Fleischmann's Diet Margarine and Ground Ginger
        (optional)
    20 fresh Cherries or 1/2 cup canned unsweetened Cherries
        (drained)
Coffee, Tea or "Free Beverage"

TOTALS:

Calories = 922
Cholesterol = 153 mg.
Sodium = 1,869 mg.

WOMEN   DAY 2

BREAKFAST:

1/2 cup unsweetened Orange Juice
1/2 Lender's Bagel (Raisin or Whole Wheat preferred)
1 tablespoon Featherweight or Dia-Mel Calorie-Reduced Jelly
   (any flavor)
Coffee or Tea with sugar substitute

LUNCH:

"Vegetable Frittata"
   1 Scrambled Egg (made with 1/4 cup Fleischmann's Egg
      Beaters Cholesterol-free egg product in 1 teaspoon
      Fleischmann's Diet Margarine)
   Topped with Fat-Free Sauteed Vegetables and Cheese as
      follows:
      1/2 cup raw Mushrooms
      1 tablespoon chopped Scallions (green onions)
      1 ounce Mozzarella Cheese (made from Skim Milk Base)
1 slice Whole Wheat Toast
1/8 fresh Honeydew Melon
Coffee, Tea or "Free Beverage"

DINNER:

1/2 cup Sugar Free JELL-O brand Diet Gelatin (any flavor)
1 (9 ounce) frozen Con Agra Light and Elegant Beef Stroganoff
   entree
1/2 cup frozen Bird's Eye Asparagus Spears (drained)
1 teaspoon Fleischmann's Diet Margarine
3/4 cup canned Del Monte Light Chunky Fruit Cocktail (drained)
Coffee, Tea or "Free Beverage"

TOTALS:

Calories = 891
Cholesterol = 118 mg.
Sodium = 1,430 mg.

WOMEN   DAY 3

BREAKFAST:

1 slice (3 ounces) frozen Weight Watchers Carrot Cake
1/2 cup Skim Milk
Coffee or Tea with sugar substitute

LUNCH:

1/2 (6 3/16-ounce package) Frozen Stouffer's Deluxe
    French Bread Pizza
"Italian Garden Salad"
    1 cup assorted greens (lettuce)
    1 tablespoon Good Season's Low-Calorie Italian Salad
        Dressing (package mix)
1 cup fresh Watermelon
Coffee, Tea or "Free Beverage"

DINNER:

"Appetizer"
    1 ounce Lite-Line Processed Cheese product (any flavor)
    2 Nabisco Low Salt Triscuit Crackers
1 frozen Budget Gourmet "Slim Line" Linguini with
    Scallops and Clams entree
1/2 cup frozen Bird's Eye chopped Spinach
1/2 ounce Sunmaid Dried Mixed Fruit Nibbles
Coffee, Tea or "Free Beverage"

TOTALS:

Calories = 913
Cholesterol = 127 mg.
Sodium = 2,239 mg.

WOMEN   DAY 4

BREAKFAST:

2 Quaker Multigrain Rice Cakes
1/2 cup Dannon Plain Low-Fat Yogurt
1/2 cup frozen or canned unsweetened Boysenberries (drained)
Coffee or Tea with sugar substitute

LUNCH:

"Cottage Cheese Fruit Plate"
    3/4 cup Lite-Line Low-Fat Cottage Cheese
    1 cup fresh/frozen unsweetened Honeydew or Cantaloupe
       Melon Balls
    1 cup fresh/frozen unsweetened Strawberries
8 Nabisco Low Salt Wheat Thin Crackers
Coffee, Tea or "Free Beverage"

DINNER:

1 cup raw shredded Cabbage on bed of Curly Endive
1 tablespoon Wish-Bone Lite Thousand Island Salad Dressing
1 teaspoon Caraway Seed (optional)
1 (3 ounce) Tyson's Chick N' Quick Breaded Chicken
    Breast Filet
12 pieces frozen Ore-Ida Lites Golden Crinkle French
    Fried Potatoes
3 tablespoons Ocean Spray Whole Berry Cranberry Sauce
1 small fresh Kiwi fruit
Coffee, Tea or "Free Beverage"

TOTALS:

Calories = 902
Cholesterol = 105 mg.
Sodium = 1,376 mg.

WOMEN DAY 5

BREAKFAST:

1 Nature Valley Oats N' Honey Granola Bar
1 cup Skim Milk
Coffee or Tea with sugar substitute

LUNCH:

1 (3 3/4 ounce) frozen Buitoni Ravioli
1 Sunkist Fruit Roll (any flavor)
Coffee, Tea or "Free Beverage"

DINNER:

1 (1 ounce) frozen Stouffer's Lean Cuisine Salisbury Steak entree
3/4 cup frozen Bird's Eye Tiny Peas
1 teaspoon Fleischmann's Diet Margarine
1/2 cup canned unsweetened Plums (drained)
Coffee, Tea or "Free Beverage"

TOTALS:

Calories = 908
Cholesterol = 189 mg.
Sodium = 1,950 mg.

WOMEN   DAY 6

BREAKFAST:

1/2 medium fresh Grapefruit (sectioned)
1 Pillsbury Toaster Corn Muffin
1/2 cup Skim Milk
Coffee or Tea with sugar substitute

LUNCH:

1 1/2 tablespoons Smucker's Natural Peanut Butter stuffed on
        2 stalks raw Celery
        1 small fresh Apple (cut in wedges)
        5 Nabisco Low Salt Triscuit Crackers
Coffee, Tea or "Free Beverage"

DINNER:

1 (8 ounce) frozen Con Agra Light and Elegant
        Glazed Chicken entree
"Vegetable Stir Fry"
        1 teaspoon Fleischmann's Diet Margarine
        1/2 cup fresh or frozen Pea Pods
        1/4 cup fresh sweet red Bell Peppers
1 small Baked Pear (prepare with sugar substitute and
        cinnamon to taste)
Coffee, Tea or "Free Beverage"

TOTALS:

Calories = 901
Cholesterol = 97 mg.
Sodium = 1,424 mg.

WOMEN   DAY 7

BREAKFAST:

1/2 cup Post or Kellogg's Corn Flakes
1/2 medium Banana
1/2 cup Skim Milk
Coffee or Tea with sugar substitute

LUNCH:

1 "Lunch Bucket" brand Lasagna or Macaroni and Beef (processed shelf-stable product)
1 cup assorted raw Vegetables including Carrots, Celery,
    Radishes and Peppers
1 medium fresh Tangerine or Nectarine
Coffee, Tea or "Free Beverage"

DINNER:

"Cranberry Apple Juice Spritzer"
    4 ounces Ocean Spray low-calorie Cranberry Apple Fruit
        Juice Drink mixed with 8 ounces no-salt added Club Soda
        or Diet Tonic Water
"Vegetables and Dip"
    1/2 cup raw Zucchini, sliced in strips
    5 small fresh Mushrooms
    4 tablespoons (2 ounces) Dean's Lite French Onion Dip
1 (9 1/2 ounce) frozen Booth Lite Fish entree with Mushroom
    Sauce and Rice
1/2 cup frozen Green Giant Brussel Sprouts
2 small fresh plums or 1/2 cup canned unsweetened plums
    (drained)
Coffee, Tea or "Free Beverage"

TOTALS:

Calories = 904
Cholesterol = 164 mg.
Sodium = 2,573 mg.

WOMEN   DAY 8

BREAKFAST:

1/3 cup unsweetened Apple Juice
2/3 cup Post or Kellogg's 40% Bran Flakes Cereal
1/2 cup Skim Milk
Coffee or Tea with sugar substitute

LUNCH:

"Phillystyle Steak Sandwich"
    1 small Kaiser or Hoagie Roll
    2 ounces cooked Roast Beef, Flank or Sirloin Steak
    2 slices of raw Onion, 2 rings Green Pepper, 2 sliced raw
        Mushrooms
    1 tablespoon Hunt's All Natural Hickory Barbeque Sauce
1/3 (5 inches across) fresh Cantaloupe Melon or 1 cup fresh/
    frozen Cantaloupe Balls
Coffee, Tea or "Free Beverage"

DINNER:

1 (7 1/4 ounce) frozen Weight Watchers Deluxe Combo Pizza
    entree
1/2 cup Sugar Free JELL-O brand Hawaiian Pineapple flavored
    gelatin
1 cup fresh or frozen unsweetened Raspberries
Coffee, Tea or "Free Beverage"

TOTALS:

Calories = 902
Cholesterol = 118 mg.
Sodium = 1,193 mg.

WOMEN   DAY 9

BREAKFAST:

3/4 cup fresh unsweetened Strawberries or Blueberries
1/4 cup Fleischmann's Egg Beaters Cholesterol-Free Egg Product
    (prepared without added fat)
1/2 Thomas Bran Toast-r-Cake
1 teaspoon Featherweight Calorie Reduced Jelly (any flavor)
Coffee or Tea with sugar substitute

LUNCH:

1/2 cup Ocean Spray Low-Calorie Cranberry Juice Cocktail
"Fisherman's Fillet"
    1 slice Dark Rye or Pumpernickel Bread
    1 frozen lightly breaded Gorton's "Light Recipe" Fish Fillet
    2 teaspoons Kraft Tartar Sauce
    2 tablespoons Vlassic canned Old Fashioned Sauerkraut
Coffee, Tea or "Free Beverage"

DINNER:

2 1/4 cups raw shredded Chinese Cabbage
(seasoned with red wine vinegar, herbs and lemon juice to taste)
1/2 cup Lipton Oriental Style Cup-A-Soup
1 (9 ounce) frozen Benihana Chicken In Spicy Garlic Sauce
    "Oriental Lite" entree
1 medium raw Orange or Tangelo
Coffee, Tea or "Free Beverage"

TOTALS:

Calories = 904
Cholesterol = 173 mg.
Sodium = 2,412 mg.

WOMEN   DAY 10

BREAKFAST:

1 frozen Aunt Jemima Blueberry Waffle
1/2 cup fresh or frozen unsweetened Blueberries
1 tablespoon Featherweight or Dia-Mel Reduced Calorie Syrup
1/2 cup Skim Milk
Coffee or Tea with sugar substitute

LUNCH:

"Nifty Nachos"
   1 ounce Lite-Line Nacho Cheese Flavored Tortilla Chips
   2 ounces Cheddar Lite-Line Reduced Calorie and Sodium
      Cheese Product (melted)
   2 tablespoons Del Monte Hot or Mild Salsa Picante Sauce
1/2 cup Libby's Lite canned Pineapple chunks (drained)
Coffee, Tea or "Free Beverage"

DINNER:

"Spaghetti and Meat Balls"
   1/2 cup cooked Prince Enriched Spaghetti
   1/2 cup Aunt Millie's Spaghetti Sauce with Sweet Peppers
      and Italian Sausage
   1 1/2 ounces ground lean beef (cooked weight) for Meat Balls
   1 tablespoon Kraft grated Parmesan Cheese
   1 1/2 inch slice of Pillsbury's Crusty French Bread Loaf
10 fresh small grapes (green or red variety)
Coffee, Tea or "Free Beverage"

TOTALS:

Calories = 908
Cholesterol = 77 mg.
Sodium = 1,601 mg.

WOMEN   DAY 11

BREAKFAST:

2/3 cup No Salt Added V-8 juice with lemon wedge
1/2 Lender's Plain or Egg Bagel
2 teaspoons Philadelphia Light Cream Cheese Spread
1 ounce Smoked Salmon (lox)
Coffee or Tea with sugar substitute

LUNCH:

"Vegetable Club Classic"
Layer Sandwich as follows:
    2 slices Whole Wheat, Rye or Pumpernickel Toast (one on top,
        one on bottom)
    1/2 cup assorted shredded Salad Greens and Alfalfa Sprouts
    1/4 medium Cucumber or Zucchini (thinly sliced)
    1 scallion (diced) and 2 radishes (sliced)
    1/2 small fresh Tomato (sliced)
    1 tablespoon Wish-Bone Lite Russian or French Dressing
1/2 cup canned unsweetened Apricots (drained)
Coffee, Tea or "Free Beverage"

DINNER:

1/2 cup frozen prepared Stouffer's New England Clam Chowder
1/2 frozen Pepperidge Farm Deli Pastry filled with Turkey, Ham
    and Cheese in Pastry
1/2 cup Bird's Eye frozen cut Green Beans
1 teaspoon Fleischmann's Diet Margarine
3/4 cup unsweetened Orange Sections (drained) or 1 medium
    fresh Orange
Coffee, Tea or "Free Beverage"

TOTALS:

Calories = 904
Cholesterol = 98 mg.
Sodium = 2,091 mg.

WOMEN   DAY 12

BREAKFAST:

2 (4-inch) Hungry Jack Extra Light Pancakes (from mix)
Topped with:
    2 teaspoons Smucker's Fruit Spread (any flavor)
1/2 cup Skim Milk
Coffee or Tea with sugar substitute

LUNCH:

1/2 cup (4 ounces) Chef Boy-Ar-Dee Beef Chili with Beans
10 Nabisco Oyster Crackers
"Salad"
    1/4 small head of Lettuce (wedge)
    1/4 cup each of chopped raw Carrot, Celery and Bell Pepper
    1 tablespoon Wish-Bone Lite Creamy Cucumber Salad
        Dressing/Lemon Wedges (as desired)
1 cup fresh Casaba Melon Balls
Coffee, Tea or "Free Beverage"

DINNER:

1 (9.25 ounces) frozen Weight Watchers Fillet of Fish
    Au Gratin entree
1 ear frozen Green Giant Nibblers Corn on the Cob
1/2 slice Dark Rye Bread
1 teaspoon Fleischmann's Diet Margarine
1 cup fresh or frozen unsweetened Raspberries,
    Blackberries or Blueberries
Coffee, Tea or "Free Beverage"

TOTALS:

Calories = 925
Cholesterol = 142 mg.
Sodium = 2,287 mg.

WOMEN   DAY 13

BREAKFAST:

1/2 cup Swiss Miss Tapioca Pudding
1 square Honey Maid Graham Cracker
1/2 cup Libby's Lite Cling Peaches (drained)
Coffee or Tea with sugar substitute

LUNCH:

6 fluid ounces Lipton's Chicken Rice Cup-A-Soup
"Pita Pocket Salad"
    1/2 Pita Pocket
    1 cup shredded Lettuce
    1 medium Carrot, grated
    1/4 medium Cucumber, diced
    1 small Tomato, sliced
    1/2 cup Chicken of the Sea low-sodium White Chunk Tuna
    1 tablespoon Kraft Light Miracle Whip Salad Dressing
5 dried Apricot halves
Coffee, Tea or "Free Beverage"

DINNER:

"Shrimp Cocktail"
    3 ounces raw or canned Shrimp (drained)
    1 tablespoon prepared Chili Sauce
1 (6 ounce) frozen pouch Chun King Chicken Chow Mein entree
1/2 cup Natural Long Grain Minute Rice
    (in individual serving pouch)
1/2 cup canned LaChoy Fancy Chinese Mixed Vegetables
    (drained)
3/4 medium raw Papaya or 1/2 medium Mango
Coffee, Tea or "Free Beverage"

TOTALS:

Calories = 912
Cholesterol = 237 mg.
Sodium = 2,310 mg.

WOMEN   DAY 14

BREAKFAST:

1/4 cup Fleischmann's Egg Beaters Cholesterol-Free Egg Product
    (prepared without added fat)
1 Pillsbury Butter Biscuit
1 teaspoon Fleischmann's Diet Margarine mixed with 1/8
    teaspoon cinnamon (optional)
1 small fresh Orange
1/2 cup Skim Milk
Coffee or Tea with sugar substitute

LUNCH:

"Open-faced Burger with the Works"
    2 ounces (cooked weight) lean Ground Beef Patty
    1/2 seeded Hamburger Bun or 1/2 Hard Roll
    2 Lettuce Leaves, 1 thin slice Sweet Onion, 2 slices fresh
        Tomato
    1 teaspoon Heinz Lite Tomato Catsup
    1 teaspoon prepared Yellow Mustard or Horseradish
12 small fresh Grapes (any variety)
Coffee, Tea or "Free Beverage"

DINNER:

1 (10 ounce) frozen Campbell's Le Menu Light Style Cheese
    Stuffed Shells with Tomato Mushroom Sauce and Broccoli
    entree
1 (3 ounce) frozen Weight Watchers Strawberry Shortcake
    topped with:
    1/2 cup fresh/frozen unsweetened Strawberries (sliced and
        mixed with sugar substitute to taste)
Coffee, Tea or "Free Beverage"

TOTALS:

Calories = 910
Cholesterol = 83 mg.
Sodium = 1,509 mg.

WOMEN   DAY 15

BREAKFAST:

1 medium fresh or dried Fig
1 cup Cheerios Cereal
1/2 cup Skim Milk
Coffee or Tea with sugar substitute

LUNCH:

"Simple Submarine Sandwich"
    1 French-style Roll
    2 slices Oscar Meyer or Louis Rich 95% to 98% Fat Free
        Luncheon Meat (any variety)
    1 slice Lite-Line Processed Cheese Product (any flavor)
    2 Lettuce Leaves, 2 fresh Tomato slices, 2 slices Bread and
        Butter Pickles
    1 teaspoon Wish-Bone Lite Italian Salad Dressing
4 small Carrot and Celery sticks
1 medium fresh Apple
Coffee, Tea or "Free Beverage"

DINNER:

1 (10 ounce) frozen Campbell's Le Menu Turkey Divan
    "Light Style" Dinner entree
1/2 frozen Green Giant Baked Potato Stuffed with Cheese topping
1 medium fresh Nectarine or Peach
Coffee, Tea or "Free Beverage"

TOTALS:

Calories = 902
Cholesterol = 126 mg.
Sodium = 2,412 mg.

WOMEN   DAY 16

BREAKFAST:

1/2 cup Quick Quaker Oats Warm Cereal topped with:
  1 teaspoon Sweet N' Low Brown Sugar Substitute (optional)
  2 tablespoons Dried Raisins
1/2 cup Skim Milk
Coffee or Tea with sugar substitute

LUNCH:

"Saucy Shrimp Pasta Salad"
  2 ounces fresh or canned (rinsed) Shrimp or Crabmeat
  1/2 cup cooked Prince Enriched Spaghetti or Macaroni
  1/4 cup fresh or frozen Cauliflower pieces
  1/4 cup fresh Bell Pepper, diced
  1/4 cup raw Broccoli pieces or steamed Asparagus spears
  1 scallion (green onion), chopped
Dressing:
  1/4 cup Dannon Plain Low-Fat Yogurt mixed with:
  1 tablespoon Lite Ranch Style Dressing
  (fresh lemon juice and herbs to taste)
1/4 cup fresh Pineapple
Coffee, Tea or "Free Beverage"

DINNER:

1/2 medium broiled Grapefruit (broil with sugar substitute
  to taste)
"Salmon/Tuna Melt"
  1 whole plain Thomas English Muffin
  1 tablespoon Kraft Light Miracle Whip Salad Dressing
  1/2 cup Alfalfa Sprouts, 5 small Mushrooms (sliced), 1 small
    Tomato (sliced)
  2 ounces flaked canned Featherweight 80% less sodium Tuna
    Fish or Salmon (drained)
  2 1/2 tablespoons prepared Cheese Sauce
Coffee, Tea or "Free Beverage"

TOTALS:

Calories = 906
Cholesterol = 138 mg.
Sodium = 1,015 mg.

WOMEN   DAY 17

BREAKFAST:

1/2 Thomas Honey Wheat or English Muffin
2 teaspoons Philadelphia Light Cream Cheese Spread
1 teaspoon Smucker's Fruit Spread (any flavor)
1/2 cup fresh or frozen unsweetened Blackberries
1/2 cup Skim Milk
Coffee or Tea with sugar substitute

LUNCH:

2 frozen Van de Kamp's Beef Enchiladas
1/2 cup canned Old El Paso Refried Beans
1 medium fresh Peach or 1/2 cup unsweetened canned
    Peaches (drained)
Coffee, Tea or "Free Beverage"

DINNER:

"Raw Spinach Salad"
    1 cup raw Spinach
    1/2 cup canned LaChoy Chop Suey Vegetables (drained)
    1/2 cup canned Del Monte No Salt Added Beets (sliced and
        drained)
    2 tablespoons Wish-Bone Lite Sweet N' Spicy French Style
        Salad Dressing
1 (11 ounce) frozen Armour Turkey Parmesan Classic Lites entree
2 dried Apple Rings
Coffee, Tea or "Free Beverage"

TOTALS:

Calories = 918
Cholesterol = 132 mg.
Sodium = 2,544 mg.

WOMEN   DAY 18

BREAKFAST:

1/2 cup Dannon Plain Low-Fat Yogurt with any of the following additions:
> 1/2 cup fresh or frozen berries (any kind) or 1 tablespoon Smucker's Fruit Spread (use sugar substitute to taste)

2 plain Nabisco Graham Crackers
Coffee or Tea with sugar substitute

LUNCH:

"Wild Turkey Salad"
> 2 ounces (cooked weight) Turkey Breast (chunks) mixed with:
> 1/2 cup frozen prepared Green Giant Long Grain White and Wild Rice (one of the Giant's "Rice Originals" line)
> 1/4 cup each of raw chopped Celery, Green Pepper and Radishes (1 Scallion optional)
> 1 tablespoon Hellman's Lite Mayonnaise

1/2 cup canned unsweetened Mandarin Orange Sections (drained)
Coffee, Tea or "Free Beverage"

DINNER:

1/2 cup Campbell's Won Ton Soup
1 (8 5/8-ounces) frozen Stouffer's Lean Cuisine Oriental Beef with Vegetables and Rice
1/2 cup canned unsweetened Del Monte Light Crushed Pineapple or Pineapple Tidbits
2 Nabisco Nilla Vanilla Wafers
Coffee, Tea or "Free Beverage"

TOTALS:

Calories = 909
Cholesterol = 191 mg.
Sodium = 2,502 mg.

WOMEN   DAY 19

BREAKFAST:

1/4 cup unsweetened Grape Juice
1 1/2 slices frozen Eggo French Toast
1 tablespoon Featherweight Low-Calorie Syrup
1/2 cup Skim Milk
Coffee or Tea with sugar substitute

LUNCH:

"Picnicking"
  1/2 container (3 1/2 ounces) Carnation's Spreadables (Turkey
      or Chicken Salad Spreadables)
  6 Nabisco Wheatsworth Crackers
"Fresh Fruit Salad"
  1/2 small Orange (sectioned)
  1/2 cup Melon (any variety)
  2-3 medium fresh or frozen unsweetened Strawberries
Coffee, Tea or "Free Beverage"

DINNER:

1 (9 5/8 ounces) frozen Stouffer's Lean Cuisine
    Beef and Pork Cannelloni with Mornay Sauce
4 ounce single serving frozen Stokely's Mixed Vegetables
1 medium Baked Apple (prepared with sugar substitute and
    cinnamon to taste)
Coffee, Tea or "Free Beverage"

TOTALS:

Calories = 923
Cholesterol = 202 mg.
Sodium = 1,980 mg.

WOMEN   DAY 20

BREAKFAST:

1 Thomas Toast-r-Cake (Bran, Blueberry or Corn)
1 teaspoon Fleischmann's Diet Margarine
Coffee or Tea with sugar substitute

LUNCH:

2 ounces (cooked weight) lean shaved Pork Tenderloin or
    2 ounces Eckrich "Calorie Watcher" Canadian Style Bacon
1/2 Large Hard Roll
1/2 cup shredded Cabbage Dressed with 1 tablespoon Durkee,
    Weight Watchers or Dia-Mel Slaw Dressing
1/2 cup Mott's Natural Style Applesauce
Coffee, Tea or "Free Beverage"

DINNER:

1 (11 ounce) frozen Stouffer's Lean Cuisine Zucchini Lasagna
    entree
1 Pillsbury Soft Breadstick
1 teaspoon Fleischmann's Diet Margarine
3/4 cup fresh Pineapple
Coffee, Tea or "Free Beverage"

TOTALS:

Calories = 876
Cholesterol = 115 mg.
Sodium = 2,700 mg.

WOMEN   DAY 21

BREAKFAST:

1 1/2 cups Quaker Puffed Rice or Puffed Wheat
1/2 cup Skim Milk
1/2 cup canned Del Monte Lite Pears (drained)
Coffee or Tea with sugar substitute

LUNCH:

"Cajun Chicken Breast"
 2 ounces (cooked weight) Chicken Breast Filet (seasoned
  with dash of spicy red sauce or cajun seasoning and
  broiled)
"Raw Rainbow Salad" (eaten raw or steamed without added fat)
 1/2 cup raw Broccoli pieces
 1/2 cup raw Cauliflower pieces
 1/2 cup raw shredded red Cabbage
 1 tablespoon Reduced Calorie Hidden Valley Ranch Salad
  Dressing
2 Ry Krisp Crackers (sesame, seasoned or natural flavor)
1/2 cup canned unsweetened Pink or White Grapefruit sections
 (drained)
Coffee, Tea or "Free Beverage"

DINNER:

1 small whole fresh Tomato (sliced), seasoned with ground
 Tarragon or sweet Basil
1 tablespoon Wish-Bone Lite Russian Salad Dressing
3/4 cup prepared Kraft Velveeta Shells and Cheese Dinner
1/2 cup frozen Green Giant's Early June Peas
1/2 cup Libby's Lite Fruit Cocktail (drained)
Coffee, Tea or "Free Beverage"

TOTALS:

Calories = 909
Cholesterol = 118 mg.
Sodium = 2,487 mg.

MEN   DAY 1

BREAKFAST:

4 "Bite Size" Sunsweet Pitted Prunes
1 Sara Lee All Butter Croissant
1 teaspoon Fleischmann's Diet Margarine
1 cup Skim Milk
Coffee or Tea with sugar substitute

LUNCH:

"Stuffed Baked Potato"
    1 medium Plain Baked Potato topped with:
        1/2 cup raw Broccoli pieces
        1/2 cup sliced Mushrooms
        1 tablespoon minced raw Onion
        3/4 cup Lite-Line Low-Fat Cottage Cheese
        1/2 small Tomato, diced
        1 tablespoon Kraft Bacon & Tomato Reduced-Calorie
          Salad Dressing
"Fruit Salad"
    1/2 cup mixed raw unsweetened Melon Balls (any melon)
    1/4 cup canned unsweetened Pineapple Chunks (drained)
    1/4 cup canned unsweetened Peaches (sliced, drained)
Coffee, Tea or "Free Beverage"

DINNER:

1 (10 ounce) Frozen Banquet Green Pepper Steak entree
1/2 cup plain baked Acorn, Butternut or Hubbard Squash topped
    with:
    1 teaspoon Fleischmann's Diet Margarine and Ground Ginger
      (optional)
1 slice Rye or Whole Grain Bread
1 teaspoon Fleischmann's Diet Margarine
20 fresh Cherries or 1/2 cup canned unsweetened Cherries
    (drained)
Coffee, Tea or "Free Beverage"

TOTALS:

Calories = 1,218
Cholesterol = 165 mg.
Sodium = 2,526 mg.

MEN   DAY 2

BREAKFAST:

1/2 cup unsweetened Orange Juice
1/2 Lender's Bagel (Raisin or Whole Wheat preferred)
1 teaspoon Fleischmann's Diet Margarine
1 tablespoon Featherweight Calorie Reduced Jelly (any flavor)
1 cup Skim Milk
Coffee or Tea with sugar substitute

LUNCH:

"Vegetable Frittata"
    2 Scrambled Eggs (made with 1/2 cup Fleischmann's Egg
        Beaters Cholesterol-Free Egg Product in 1 teaspoon
        Fleischmann's Diet Margarine)
Topped with Fat Free Sauteed Vegetables and Cheese as follows:
    1/2 cup raw Mushrooms (sliced)
    1 tablespoon chopped Scallions (green onions)
    1 ounce Mozzarella Cheese (made from Skim Milk Base)
    * (chopped Chives and Parsley optional)
2 slices Whole Wheat Toast with 2 teaspoons Fleischmann's
    Diet Margarine
1/8 or 1 cup fresh Honeydew Melon
Coffee, Tea or "Free Beverage"

DINNER:

1 (9 ounce) frozen Con Agra Light and Elegant
    Beef Stroganoff entree
1 cup frozen Bird's Eye Asparagus Spears (drained)
1 teaspoon Fleischmann's Diet Margarine
1/2 cup JELL-O Sugar-Free Vanilla Pudding (made with Skim
    Milk)
1 cup canned Del Monte Light Chunky Fruit Cocktail (drained)
Coffee, Tea or "Free Beverage"

TOTALS:

Calories = 1,219
Cholesterol = 138 mg.
Sodium = 2,190 mg.

MEN   DAY 3

BREAKFAST:

1 slice (3 ounces) frozen Weight Watchers Carrot Cake
1/2 medium raw Apple (in wedges)
1 cup Skim Milk
Coffee or Tea with sugar substitute

LUNCH:

3/4 (6 3/16-ounce package) Frozen Stouffer's Deluxe French Bread
    Pizza
"Italian Garden Salad"
    1 cup assorted Greens (any type lettuce)
    1 tablespoon Good Season's Low-Calorie Italian Salad
        Dressing (package mix)
1 1/2 cups fresh Watermelon
Coffee, Tea or "Free Beverage"

DINNER:

"Appetizer"
    1 ounce Lite-Line Processed Cheese Product (any flavor)
    4 Nabisco Low Salt Triscuit Crackers
1 frozen Budget Gourmet "Slim Line" Linguini with Scallops and
    Clams entree
1/2 cup frozen Bird's Eye chopped Spinach (drained)
1 teaspoon Fleischmann's Diet Margarine
1 ounce Sunmaid Dried Mixed Fruit Nibbles
Coffee, Tea or "Free Beverage"

TOTALS:

Calories = 1,221
Cholesterol = 147 mg.
Sodium = 2,661 mg.

MEN   DAY 4

BREAKFAST:

2 Quaker Multigrain Rice Cakes
1 tablespoon Skippy Super Chunk Peanut Butter
3/4 cup Dannon Plain Low-Fat Yogurt
1/2 cup frozen or canned unsweetened Boysenberries (drained)
Coffee or Tea with sugar substitute

LUNCH:

"Cottage Cheese Fruit Plate"
    3/4 cup Lite-Line Low Fat Cottage Cheese
    1 1/2 cups fresh/frozen unsweetened Honeydew or
        Cantaloupe Melon Balls
    1 cup fresh/frozen unsweetened Strawberries
15 Nabisco Low Salt Wheat Thin Crackers
Coffee, Tea or "Free Beverage"

DINNER:

"Salad"
    1 cup raw shredded Cabbage on bed of Curly Endive
    1/2 medium Cucumber (sliced)
    1/2 small Tomato (sliced)
    1/4 cup fresh/frozen Peas
    1 tablespoon Wish-Bone Lite Thousand Island Salad Dressing
    *Lemon, fresh herbs and Caraway seed (optional)
1 (3 ounce) Tyson's Chick N' Quick Breaded Chicken Breast Filet
12 pieces frozen Ore-Ida Lites Golden Crinkle French Fries
1/4 cup Ocean Spray Whole Berry Cranberry Sauce
1 small fresh Kiwi fruit
Coffee, Tea or "Free Beverage"

TOTALS:

Calories = 1,216
Cholesterol = 77 mg.
Sodium = 1,525 mg.

MEN   DAY 5

BREAKFAST:

1 Nature Valley Oats N' Honey Granola Bar
1 cup Del Monte Light Chunky Fruit Cocktail (drained)
1 cup Skim Milk
Coffee or Tea with sugar substitute

LUNCH:

1 (3 3/4 ounce) frozen Buitoni Ravioli
1 Sunkist Fruit Roll (any flavor)
5 small Gingersnaps
Coffee, Tea or "Free Beverage"

DINNER:

"Mock Bloody Mary"
    2/3 cup No Salt Added V-8 or Tomato Juice
    Tabasco Sauce and Celery Seed to taste (optional)
    2 stalks Celery
1 (9 1/2 ounce) frozen Stouffer's Lean Cuisine
    Salisbury Steak entree
1/2 cup frozen Bird's Eye Cut Green Beans
1 small enriched Hard Roll
1 teaspoon Fleischmann's Diet Margarine
1 medium fresh Orange or Nectarine
Coffee, Tea of "Free Beverage"

TOTALS:

Calories = 1,226
Cholesterol = 189 mg.
Sodium = 1,780 mg.

MEN   DAY 6

BREAKFAST:

1 small whole Grapefruit (halved & sectioned)
1 Pillsbury Toaster Corn Muffin
2 teaspoon Featherweight Calorie Reduced Jelly (any flavor)
1 cup Skim Milk
Coffee or Tea with sugar substitute

LUNCH:

"Grape Bubbly"
    1/2 cup Minute Maid Light N' Juicy Grape Drink mixed with 6
        ounces Club Soda
2 tablespoons Smucker's Natural Peanut Butter stuffed on:
    3 stalks raw Celery (in sticks)
    1 small raw Carrot (in sticks)
    1 small raw Apple (in sections)
    1/2 Lender's Raisin N' Honey Bagel
Coffee, Tea or "Free Beverage"

DINNER:

1 (8 ounce) frozen Con Agra Light and Elegant
    Glazed Chicken entree
"Vegetable Stir Fry"
    1 teaspoon Fleischmann's Diet Margarine
    1/2 cup fresh or frozen Pea Pods
    1/2 cup fresh sweet red Bell Pepper
    Low Sodium Broth and Herbs to taste (optional)
1 small Baked Pear (prepared with sugar substitute and
    cinnamon to taste)
1/2 cup Edy's Grand Light Strawberry or Vanilla Ice Cream
Coffee, Tea or "Free Beverage"

TOTALS:

Calories = 1,206
Cholesterol = 125 mg.
Sodium = 1,522 mg.

MEN   DAY 7

BREAKFAST:

1 cup Post or Kellogg's 40% Bran Flakes
1/2 medium raw Banana
1 cup Skim Milk
Coffee or Tea with sugar substitute

LUNCH:

1 "Lunch Bucket" brand Lasagna or Macaroni and Beef
   (processed shelf stable product)
1 cup assorted raw Vegetables including Carrots, Celery,
   Radishes and Peppers
1 tablespoon Reduced Calorie Salad Dressing (any variety)
Red Wine Vinegar and Lemon Wedge (optional)
1 medium fresh Tangerine or Nectarine
1/2 cup frozen Low-Fat Yogurt (any brand, any flavor)
Coffee, Tea or "Free Beverage"

DINNER:

"Cranberry Apple Juice Spritzer"
    1/2 cup Ocean Spray low-calorie Cranberry Apple Fruit Juice
       Drink mixed with 8 ounces no salt added Club Soda or
       Diet Tonic Water
1 (9 1/2 ounce) frozen Booth Lite Fish entree with Mushroom
   Sauce and Rice
1/2 cup frozen Green Giant Brussel Sprouts
1 small Dinner Roll
2 teaspoons Fleischmann's Diet Margarine
2 small fresh Plums or 1/2 cup canned unsweetened Plums
   (drained)
Coffee, Tea or "Free Beverage"

TOTALS

Calories = 1,208
Cholesterol = 158 mg.
Sodium = 3,000 mg.

MEN   DAY 8

BREAKFAST:

1/3 cup unsweetened Apple Juice
1 cup Kellogg's or Post Corn Flakes
1 slice Whole Grain Toast
1 teaspoon Featherweight or Dia-Mel Calorie Reduced Jelly
     (any flavor)
1 cup Skim Milk
Coffee or Tea with sugar substitute

LUNCH:

"Phillystyle Steak Sandwich"
     1 large Kaiser or Hoagie Roll
     3 ounces (cooked weight) Roast Beef, Flank or Sirloin Steak
     2 slices of raw Onion, 2 rings Green Pepper, 2 sliced raw
          Mushrooms
     1 tablespoon Hunt's All Natural Hickory Barbeque Sauce
1/3 (5 inches across) fresh Cantaloupe Melon or 1 cup fresh/
     frozen Cantaloupe Balls
Coffee, Tea or "Free Beverage"

DINNER:

"Italian Salad"
     2 cups assorted Lettuce (any variety)
     1/2 medium Zucchini or Cucumber (sliced)
     2 large Lindsay Ripe Olives
     2 tablespoons Good Season's Low Calorie Italian Salad
          Dressing
     (red wine vinegar, herbs and lemon juice to taste)
1 (7 1/4 ounces) frozen Weight Watchers Deluxe Combo Pizza
     entree
1 cup fresh or frozen unsweetened Raspberries
1/2 cup Sugar-Free JELL-O brand Hawaiian Pineapple flavored
     gelatin
Coffee, Tea or "Free Beverage"

TOTALS:

Calories = 1,212
Cholesterol = 143 mg.
Sodium = 2,008 mg.

MEN   DAY 9

BREAKFAST:

1/2 cup Apple, Orange or Pineapple Juice
2 Scrambled Eggs (prepared with 1/2 cup Fleischmann's Egg-
    Beaters Cholesterol-Free Egg Product and 1 teaspoon
    Fleischmann's Diet Margarine)
1 Thomas Bran Toast-r-Cake
1 teaspoon Featherweight Calorie Reduced Jelly (any flavor)
1 teaspoon Fleischmann's Diet Margarine
Coffee or Tea with sugar substitute

LUNCH:

2/3 cup Ocean Spray Low-Calorie Cranberry Juice Cocktail
"Fisherman's Fillet"
    2 slices Dark Rye or Pumpernickel Bread
    1 frozen lightly breaded Gorton's "Light Recipe" Fish Fillet
    2 teaspoons Kraft Tartar Sauce
    2 tablespoons Vlassic canned Old Fashioned Sauerkraut
1/2 cup Mott's Natural Style Apple Sauce
Coffee, Tea or "Free Beverage"

DINNER:

2 1/4 cups raw shredded Chinese Cabbage
1 1/2 tablespoons Henri's Sweet N' Tart Salad Dressing
1/2 cup Lipton Oriental Style Cup-A-Soup
1 (9 ounce) frozen Benihana Chicken in Spicy Garlic Sauce
    "Oriental Lite" entree
1 medium raw Orange and Tangelo
Coffee, Tea or "Free Beverage"

TOTALS:
Calories = 1,215
Cholesterol = 160 mg.
Sodium = 2,752 mg.

MEN   DAY 10

BREAKFAST:

2 frozen Aunt Jemima Blueberry Waffles
1/2 cup fresh or frozen unsweetened Blueberries
1 tablespoon Featherweight or Dia-Mel Reduced Calorie Syrup
1 cup Skim Milk
Coffee or Tea with sugar substitute

LUNCH:

"Nifty Nachos"
    1 ounce Lite-Line Nacho Cheese Flavored Tortilla Chips
    3 ounces Cheddar Lite-Line Reduced Calorie and Sodium
        Cheese Product (melted)
    2 tablespoons Del Monte Hot or Mild Salsa Picante Sauce
1/4 cup prepared Betty Crocker's "Suddenly Salad Mix"
    (any variety)
1/2 cup Libby's Lite canned Pineapple Chunks (drained)
Coffee, Tea or "Free Beverage"

DINNER:

"Spaghetti and Meat Balls"
    3/4 cup cooked Prince Enriched Spaghetti
    1/2 cup Aunt Millie's Spaghetti Sauce with Sweet Peppers
        and Italian Sausage
    1 1/2 ounces (cooked weight) lean Ground Beef for Meat Balls
    1 tablespoon Kraft grated Parmesan Cheese
1 1/2 inch slice of Pillsbury's Crusty French Bread Loaf
12 fresh small Grapes (green or red variety)
Coffee, Tea or "Free Beverage"

TOTALS:

Calories = 1,225
Cholesterol = 95 mg.
Sodium = 2,177 mg.

MEN   DAY 11

BREAKFAST:

2/3 cup No Salt Added V-8 Juice with Lemon Wedge
1/2 Lender's Plain or Egg Bagel
1 tablespoon Philadelphia Light Cream Cheese Spread
1 ounce Smoked Salmon (lox)
2 medium fresh or 1/2 cup canned unsweetened Plums (drained)
Coffee or Tea with sugar substitute

LUNCH:

"Vegetable Club Classic"
Layer sandwich as follows:
    2 slices Whole Wheat, Rye or Pumpernickel Toast (one on top,
       one on bottom)
    1/2 cup assorted shredded Salad Greens and Alfalfa Sprouts
    1/4 medium Cucumber or Zucchini (thinly sliced)
    1 scallion (diced) and 2 radishes (sliced)
    1 small Tomato (sliced)
    1 1/2 tablespoons Wish-Bone Lite Russian or French Dressing
1 cup canned unsweetened Apricots (drained)
Coffee, Tea or "Free Beverage"

DINNER:

1 frozen Pepperidge Farm Deli filled with Turkey, Ham and
    Cheese in Pastry
3/4 cup frozen Bird's Eye Green Beans with Corn, Carrots and
    Pearl Onions
1 teaspoon Fleischmann's Diet Margarine
1 cup fresh or canned unsweetened Pineapple Chunks (drained)
Coffee, Tea or "Free Beverage"

TOTALS:

Calories = 1,211
Cholesterol = 152 mg.
Sodium = 2,544 mg.

MEN   DAY 12

BREAKFAST:

2 (4-inch) Hungry Jack Extra Light Pancakes (from mix)
   topped with:
   1 cup fresh/frozen unsweetened Strawberries mixed with
      sugar substitute to taste
1 ounce Grilled Louis Rich Turkey Ham (prepared without
   added fat)
1 cup Skim Milk
Coffee or Tea with sugar substitute

LUNCH:

3/4 cup Chef Boy-Ar-Dee Beef Chili with Beans
10 Nabisco Oyster Crackers
"Super Salad"
   1/4 small Head of Lettuce (in wedge)
   1/4 cup each of chopped raw Carrot, Cauliflower, Celery and
      Bell Pepper
   1 tablespoon Wish-Bone Lite Creamy Cucumber Salad
      Dressing and Lemon Wedges as desired
1 cup raw Casaba Melon Balls
Coffee, Tea or "Free Beverage"

DINNER:

1 (9.25 ounces) frozen Weight Watchers Fillet of Fish
   Au Gratin entree
2 ears frozen Green Giant "Nibblers" Corn on the Cob
1/2 slice dark Rye or Pumpernickel Bread
2 teaspoons Fleischmann's Diet Margarine
1 cup fresh or frozen unsweetened Raspberries,
   Blackberries or Blueberries
Coffee, Tea or "Free Beverage"

TOTALS:

Calories = 1,215
Cholesterol = 188 mg.
Sodium = 2,968 mg.

MEN   DAY 13

BREAKFAST:

1/2 cup Swiss Miss Tapioca Pudding
2 squares Honey Maid Graham Crackers
1 cup Libby's Lite Cling Peaches (drained)
Coffee or Tea with sugar substitute

LUNCH:

6 fluid ounces Lipton's Chicken Rice Cup-A-Soup
"Pita Pocket Salad"
    1/2 Pita Pocket
    1 cup shredded Lettuce
    1 medium Carrot, grated
    1/4 medium Cucumber, diced
    1 small Tomato, sliced
    1/4 cup Bush's Best Light Red Kidney Beans
        (canned, drained)
    1/2 cup Chicken of the Sea low-sodium White Chunk Tuna
    1 1/2 tablespoons Kraft Light Miracle Whip Salad Dressing
3 dried Apricot halves
Coffee, Tea or "Free Beverage"

DINNER:

"Shrimp Cocktail"
    4 ounces raw or canned Shrimp (drained)
    1 tablespoon prepared Chili Sauce
1 (6 ounce) frozen pouch Chun King Chicken Chow Mein entree
3/4 cup Natural Long Grain Minute Rice
3/4 cup canned LaChoy Fancy Chinese Mixed Vegetables
    (drained)
3/4 medium raw Papaya or 1/2 medium Mango
5 Nilla Vanilla Wafers
Coffee, Tea or "Free Beverage"

TOTALS:
Calories = 1,212
Cholesterol = 259 mg.
Sodium = 2,572 mg.

MEN DAY 14

BREAKFAST:

2 Pillsbury Butter Biscuits
1 tablespoon Fleischmann's Diet Margarine mixed
    with 1/8 teaspoon cinnamon (optional)
1 medium fresh Orange
1 cup Skim Milk
Coffee or Tea with sugar substitute

LUNCH:

"Open-faced Burger with the Works"
    1 whole seeded Hamburger Bun or 1 whole Hard Roll
    3 ounces (cooked weight) lean Ground Beef Patty
    2 Lettuce Leaves, 1 thin Slice Sweet Onion, 2 slices fresh
        Tomato
    1 teaspoon Heinz Lite Tomato Catsup
    1 teaspoon prepared Yellow Mustard or Horseradish
24 small fresh Grapes (any variety)
Coffee, Tea or "Free Beverage"

DINNER:

"Raw Spinach Salad"
    2 cups raw Spinach Greens
    3 medium Radishes
    2 medium Scallions
    Fresh Lemon and Red Wine Vinegar (optional)
    2 teaspoons Bacos
1 (10 ounce) frozen Campbell's Le Menu Light Style Cheese
    stuffed Shells with Tomato Mushroom Sauce and
    Broccoli entree
1 slice Whole Wheat Bread
2 teaspoons Fleischmann's Diet Margarine
1 cup fresh or frozen unsweetened Berries (any kind)
Coffee, Tea or "Free Beverage"

TOTALS:

Calories = 1,215
Cholesterol = 133 mg.
Sodium = 2,113 mg.

MEN   DAY 15

BREAKFAST:

1 1/4 cup Cheerios Cereal
1 1/2 cup fresh/frozen unsweetened Raspberries
1 slice Fresh Horizons Bread (any variety)
1 teaspoon Fleischmann's Diet Margarine
1 cup Skim Milk
Coffee or Tea with sugar substitute

LUNCH:

"Simple Submarine Sandwich"
    1 French-style Roll
    2 slices Oscar Meyer or Louis Rich 95% to 98% Fat Free
        Luncheon Meat (any variety)
    1 slice Lite-Line Processed Cheese Product (any flavor)
    2 Lettuce Leaves, 2 fresh Tomato slices
    1 teaspoon Wish-Bone Lite Italian Salad Dressing
1/2 cup canned Green Giant Three Bean Salad (drained)
1 medium fresh Apple
Coffee, Tea or "Free Beverage"

DINNER:

1 (10 ounce) frozen Campbell's Le Menu Turkey Divan
    "Light Style" Dinner entree
1/2 cup Uncle Ben's Brown and Wild Rice (Mushroom Recipe Mix)
1/2 cup fresh cooked Carrots (plain)
2 teaspoons Fleischmann's Diet Margarine
1 medium fresh Nectarine or Peach
Coffee, Tea or "Free Beverage"

TOTALS:

Calories = 1,208
Cholesterol = 137 mg.
Sodium = 3,315 mg.

MEN   DAY 16

BREAKFAST:

1 1/4 cup Quick Quaker Oats Warm Cereal topped with:
    1 teaspoon Sweet N' Low Brown Sugar Substitute (optional)
    2 tablespoons Dried Raisins
1/2 cup Skim Milk
Coffee or Tea with sugar substitute

LUNCH:

"Saucy Shrimp Pasta Salad"
    2 ounces fresh or canned (drained) Shrimp or Crabmeat
    1/2 cup cooked Prince Enriched Spaghetti or Macaroni
    1/4 cup fresh or frozen Cauliflower pieces
    1/4 cup fresh Bell Pepper, diced
    1/4 cup raw Broccoli pieces or steamed Asparagus Spears
    1 Scallion (green onion), chopped
Dressing:
1/4 cup Dannon Plain Low-Fat Yogurt mixed with:
    2 tablespoons Lite Ranch Style Dressing
    (fresh lemon juice, grated Parsley and herbs to taste)
3/4 cup fresh or 1/3 cup canned unsweetened Pineapple (drained)
Coffee, Tea or "Free Beverage"

DINNER:

1/2 medium broiled Grapefruit (broil with sugar substitute to
    taste)
"Salmon/Tuna Melt"
    1 whole plain Thomas English Muffin
    1 tablespoon Kraft Light Miracle Whip Salad Dressing
    1/2 cup Alfalfa Sprouts, 5 small Mushrooms (sliced), 1 small
        Tomato (sliced)
    4 ounces flaked canned Featherweight 80% less sodium Tuna
        Fish or Salmon (drained)
    2 1/2 tablespoons prepared Cheese Sauce
1/2 cup Borden's Lemon, Orange or Rainbow Sherbet
Coffee, Tea or "Free Beverage"

TOTALS:

Calories = 1,213
Cholesterol = 201 mg.
Sodium = 992 mg.

MEN   DAY 17

BREAKFAST:

1 whole Thomas Honey Wheat or English Muffin
1 tablespoon Philadelphia Light Cream Cheese Spread
1 tablespoon Smucker's Fruit Spread (any flavor)
1/2 cup fresh or frozen unsweetened Blackberries
1 cup Skim Milk
Coffee or Tea with sugar substitute

LUNCH:

1 frozen Van de Kamp's Beef Enchiladas
1/2 cup canned Old El Paso Refried Beans
1 medium fresh Peach or 1/2 cup unsweetened canned Peaches
    (drained)
1 Nabisco Almost Home Oatmeal Raisin Cookie
Coffee, Tea or "Free Beverage"

DINNER:

"Raw Spinach Salad"
    2 cups raw Spinach
    1/2 cup canned LaChoy Chop Suey Vegetables (drained)
    1/2 cup canned Del Monte No Salt Added Beets (sliced and
        drained)
    2 tablespoons Wish-Bone Lite Sweet N' Spicy French Style
        Salad Dressing
1 (10 ounce) frozen Le Menu Chicken Cacciatore entree
4 pieces Melba Toast (any variety)
1 teaspoon Fleischmann's Diet Margarine
3 dried Apple Rings
Coffee, Tea or "Free Beverage"

TOTALS:

Calories = 1,218
Cholesterol = 161 mg.
Sodium = 2,983 mg.

MEN   DAY 18

BREAKFAST:

1 cup Dannon Plain Low-Fat Yogurt with any kind of the
    following additions:
        1 cup fresh or frozen berries (any kind) or 2 tablespoons
            Smucker's Fruit Spread (use sugar substitute to taste)
3 plain Nabisco Graham Crackers
Coffee or Tea with sugar substitute

LUNCH:

"Wild Turkey Salad"
        2 ounces (cooked weight) Turkey Breast (chunks) mixed
            with:
        1/2 cup frozen prepared Green Giant Long Grain White and
            Wild Rice (one of the Giant's "Rice Originals" line)
        1/4 cup each of raw chopped Celery, Green Pepper and
            Radishes (1 Scallion optional)
        1 tablespoon Hellman's Light Mayonnaise
1 cup canned unsweetened Mandarin Orange Sections (drained)
Coffee, Tea or "Free Beverage"

DINNER:

1/2 cup Campbell's Won Ton Soup
1 (8 5/8 ounces) frozen Stouffer's Lean Cuisine Oriental Beef with
    Vegetables and Rice
1/4 cup canned Chow Mein Fried Noodles
3 medium fresh Apricots or 1 Dried Fig
2 Nabisco Almond Windmill Cookies
Coffee, Tea or "Free Beverage"

TOTALS:

Calories = 1,202
Cholesterol = 193 mg.
Sodium = 2,735 mg.

MEN   DAY 19

BREAKFAST:

1/3 cup unsweetened Grape or Prune Juice
2 slices frozen Eggo French Toast
1 tablespoon Featherweight Low-Calorie Syrup
1 cup Skim Milk
Coffee or Tea with sugar substitute

LUNCH:

"Picnicking"
    1/2 container (3 1/2 ounces) Carnation's Spreadables (Chicken
       or Turkey Salad Spreadables)
    8 Nabisco Wheatsworth Crackers
"Fresh Fruit Salad"
    1 small Orange (sectioned)
    1/2 cup assorted Melon Balls (any variety)
    6 medium fresh or frozen unsweetened Strawberries
1 frozen JELL-O brand Gelatin Pop (any flavor)
Coffee, Tea or "Free Beverage"

DINNER:

1 (9 5/8 ounces) frozen Stouffer's Lean Cuisine Beef and Pork
    Cannelloni with Mornay Sauce
1 (4 ounces) single serving frozen Stokely's Mixed Vegetables
2 Bread Sticks (4 inches long by 1 inch thick) any variety
1 teaspoon Fleischmann's Diet Margarine
1 medium Baked Apple (prepared with sugar substitute and
    cinnamon to taste)
Coffee, Tea or "Free Beverage"

TOTALS:

Calories = 1,218
Cholesterol = 210 mg.
Sodium = 2,353 mg.

MEN DAY 20

BREAKFAST:

2 Nabisco Shredded Wheat Biscuits
1/2 medium Banana
1 cup Skim Milk
Coffee or Tea with sugar substitute

LUNCH:

"Shaved Pork Sandwich"
  2 ounces (cooked weight) lean shaved Pork Tenderloin or 2
    ounces Eckrich "Calorie Watcher" Canadian Style Bacon
  1 large Hard Roll
  1 tablespoon Heinz Barbeque Sauce (any variety)
1/2 cup shredded Cabbage dressed with 1 tablespoon Kraft
  Coleslaw Dressing
1/2 cup Mott's Natural Style Applesauce
Coffee, Tea or "Free Beverage"

DINNER:

"Salad"
  1/4 medium head lettuce
  1/4 cup seasoned Croutons, 3 small or 2 large Lindsay
    Ripe Olives
  1 tablespoon Kraft Reduced Calorie Salad Dressing
    (any variety)
1 (11 ounce) frozen Stouffer's Lean Cuisine Zucchini
  Lasagna entree
1 (3 fluid ounce) Yoplait Cherry Soft Frozen Yogurt Bar
12 whole fresh or frozen unsweetened Cherries
Coffee, Tea or "Free Beverage"

TOTALS:

Calories = 1,228
Cholesterol = 113 mg.
Sodium = 2,172 mg.

MEN   DAY 21

BREAKFAST:

1 Hostess Crumb Cake
1 1/2 cups Quaker Puffed Rice or Puffed Wheat Cereal
1/2 cup Skim Milk
1/2 cup canned Del Monte Lite Pears (drained)
Coffee or Tea with sugar substitute

LUNCH:

"Cajun Chicken Breast"
>   3 ounces (cooked weight) Chicken Breast Filet (seasoned
>   with dash of spicy red sauce or cajun seasoning and
>   broiled)

"Raw Rainbow Salad" (eaten raw or steamed without added fat)
>   1/2 cup raw Broccoli pieces
>   1/2 cup raw Cauliflower pieces
>   1/2 cup shredded Red Cabbage
>   1 tablespoon Reduced Calorie Hidden Valley Ranch Salad
>   Dressing

2 Ry Krisp Crackers (sesame, seasoned or natural flavor)
1 cup unsweetened Pink or White Grapefruit sections (drained)
Coffee, Tea or "Free Beverage"

DINNER:

1 small whole fresh Tomato (sliced), seasoned with ground
    Tarragon or Sweet Basil
1 tablespoon Wish-Bone Lite Russian Salad Dressing
1 cup prepared Kraft Velveeta Shells and Cheese Dinner
1/2 cup frozen Green Giant's Early June Peas
1/2 cup Libby's Lite Fruit Cocktail (drained)
Coffee, Tea or "Free Beverage"

TOTALS:

Calories = 1,223
Cholesterol = 190 mg.
Sodium = 1,733 mg.

Introduction to Shopping Lists

To help you follow the 21-day *Expresslane Diet,* three separate weekly shopping lists have been provided. Shopping list number one coincides with planned menus from days one through seven. Lists two and three represent days eight through fourteen and fifteen through twenty-one, respectively.

The amounts or sizes of food items have been specified for one dieter. Therefore, if you are following this diet with a partner, you need to adjust portion sizes accordingly. Before shopping, remember to check these lists against items you may have on hand in your kitchen, to avoid duplicate purchases.

You are not restricted to any brand-name products. If you are unable to find a specified brand-name item, simply refer to the exchange lists for an appropriate substitution.

Shopping List Abbreviation Key

drsg = dressing	oz = ounce
FF = fat free	pkg = package
fl = fluid	sm = small
jce = juice	unswt = unsweetened
lb = pound	w/ = with
lg = large	/ = or
med = medium	

SHOPPING LIST   WEEK 1

PRODUCE

1 sm Apple
*2 med Apples
1 med Banana
*1 med Orange
1 sm Cantaloupe/Honeydew
  Melon
1 med Grapefruit
1 sm Kiwi Fruit
1 med Lemon
1 sm Pear
1 pint Strawberries
1 med Tangerine/Nectarine
sm wedge Watermelon
1 med stalk Broccoli
1 bunch Carrots
1 sm head Cabbage
1 bunch Celery
1 med head Lettuce
1/2 lb Mushrooms
4 oz Pea Pods
1 sm Red/Yellow Pepper
1 med Baking Potato
1 bunch Scallions (green onions)
1 sm Squash
1 med Zucchini

PACKAGED GOODS

(12 oz) Sunsweet Bite Size Pitted
  Prunes
(6 oz) Sunmaid Dried Fruit Nibbles
(.75 oz) Sunkist Fruit Roll (any flavor)
(10 oz) Nature Valley Oats N'
  Honey Granola Bars
(0.3 oz) Sugar Free JELL-O Gelatin
  (any flavor)
(8 oz) tube Hungry Jack Extra Rich
  Buttermilk Biscuits
(9 1/2 oz) Nabisco Low-Salt
  Triscuit Crackers
(10 oz) Nabisco Low-Salt Wheat

Thin Crackers
(4 1/2 oz) Quaker Rice, Wheat or
  Corn Flakes
(12 oz) Kellogg's/Post Corn Flakes
(8 1/2 oz) "Lunch Bucket"
  Lasagna/Macaroni and Beef
  entree
1 package Good Season's Low
  Calorie Salad Dressing Mix
*(1.3 oz) Sugar Free JELL-O
  Vanilla Pudding
*(12 oz) pkg Gingersnaps
*1/2 gallon Minute Maid Lite 'N
  Juicy Grape Drink

DAIRY

1 lb Lite-Line Low-Fat Cottage
  Cheese
8 oz Mozzarella Cheese
12 3/4 oz Lite-Line Cheese Product
  (any flavor)
1 quart Skim Milk
1 lb Tub/Sticks Fleischmann's Diet
  Margarine
8 oz Dannon Plain Low-Fat Yogurt
8 oz Dean's Extra Light French
  Onion Dip

FROZEN FOODS

(6 oz) can unswt Orange Juice
(16 oz) pkg unswt Assorted Melon
  Balls
(12 oz) pkg unswt
  Blackberries/Blueberries
(10 oz) pkg Lender's Bagels
  (Raisin or Whole Wheat)
1 pkg Pillsbury Toaster Corn
  Muffins
(6 oz) pkg Weight Watchers Carrot
  Cake
(16 oz) pkg Fleischmann's Egg
  Beaters

(10 oz) Banquet Green Pepper Steak entree

(9 1/2 oz) Budget Gourmet Slim Line Linguini w/ Scallops and Clams entree

(11 oz) Stouffer's Lean Cuisine Salisbury Steak entree

(8 oz) Con Agra Light and Elegant Glazed Chicken entree

(9 1/2 oz) Booth Lite Fish entree w/ Mushroom Sauce and Rice

(12 oz) Tyson's Chick N' Quick Breaded Chicken Breast Filet

(6 3/16 oz) Stouffer's Deluxe French Bread Pizza entree

(3 3/4 oz) Buitoni Ravioli

(3 1/2 oz) Ore-Ida Lites Crinkle Cut French Fried Potatoes

(10 oz) pkgs each Bird's Eye Chopped Spinach, Tiny Peas and Asparagus Spears

(9 oz) Green Giant's Brussel Sprouts

*(6 oz) box Sara Lee All Butter Croissants

*2 (1 lb) pkgs unswt Assorted Melon Balls

*(10 oz) Bird's Eye Cut Green Beans

*1 quart Edy's Grand Lite Vanilla or Strawberry Ice Cream

*1 pint Low-Fat Yogurt (any fruit flavor)

BOTTLED/CANNED

10 oz Smucker's Fruit Spread (any flavor)

8 oz Featherweight Calorie Reduced Jelly (any flavor)

12 oz Smucker's Natural Peanut Butter

8 1/2 oz each unswt Cherries and Plums

8 1/2 oz Del Monte Light Chunky Fruit Cocktail

16 oz Ocean Spray Whole Berry Cranberry Sauce

8 oz Kraft Bacon & Tomato Reduced Calorie Salad drsg

8 oz Wish-Bone Lite Thousand Island Salad drsg

16 oz Vinegar (regular or herb based)

32 fl oz Ocean Spray Low-Calorie Cranberry Apple Fruit Juice drink

*16 oz Libby's Lite Fruit Cocktail

*24 fl oz No-Salt Added Tomato Juice

BAKERY/DELI

1 Loaf Catherine Clark's/Fresh Horizon's Whole Bran Bread

STAPLES

"Free Beverages" from *The Expresslane Diet*

Sugar Substitute (Sweet 'N Low) as desired (white/brown)

Low Sodium Spices and Herbs from *The Expresslane Diet*, as desired

*for men only

SHOPPING LIST

WEEK 2
(DAYS 8 - 14)

PRODUCE

1 bunch Grapes (seedless variety)
1 med Lemon
3 med Oranges
1 Papaya/Mango
1 pint Strawberries
*2 pints Strawberries
1 sm Head Cabbage
1 bag Carrots
1 bunch Celery
1 med Cucumber
1 med Head Lettuce
1/2 lb Mushrooms
2 med Green Peppers
1 sm Purple Onion
1 bunch Radishes
1 bunch Scallions (green onions)
2 sm Tomatoes
*10 oz bag Spinach Greens

PACKAGED GOODS

(16 oz) Post/Kellogg's 40% Bran
  Flakes
1 pkg Thomas Bran Toast-r-Cakes
(10 oz) Pillsbury Crusty French
  Bread
(4 1/2 oz) Pillsbury Butter Biscuits
(16 oz) Nabisco Honey Maid
  Graham Crackers
(12 oz) Oyster Crackers
(7 oz) Single Serving bags Natural
  Long Grain Minute Rice
(7 oz) Prince/Enriched Spaghetti
(2 lb) Hungry Jack Extra Light
  Pancake Mix
(1.2 oz) Lipton Oriental Style Cup-
  A-Soup Mix
(1.2 oz) Lipton Lite Chicken Rice
  Cup-A-Soup Mix
1 sm bag Lite-Line Nacho Cheese
  Flavored Tortilla Chips
(6 oz) Dried Apricot Halves

(0.3 oz) Sugar Free JELL-O Gelatin
  (any flavor)
*(6 1/4 oz) pkg Betty Crocker's
  "Suddenly Salad" Mix (any
  variety)
*(12 oz) box Nabisco Nilla Vanilla
  Wafers

DAIRY

12 3/4 oz Lite-Line Cheese Product
  (any flavor)
8 oz Tub/Sticks Fleischmann's Diet
  Margarine
8 oz Tub/Stick Philadelphia Light
  Cream Cheese
1 1/2 oz Parmesan Cheese
16 oz Swiss Miss Tapioca Pudding
  Packs
1 quart Skim Milk

FROZEN FOODS

(6 oz) unswt Apple Juice
(16 oz) pkg unswt Assorted Melon
  Balls
(12 oz) pkg unswt Red
  Raspberries
(12 oz) pkg unswt Blueberries
(16 oz) pkg Fleischmann's Egg
  Beaters
(10 oz) pkg Aunt Jemima
  Blueberry Waffles
(10 oz) Lender's Bagels (Plain/Egg)
(12 oz) pkg Pita Pockets
(7 1/4 oz) Weight Watchers Deluxe
  Combo Pizza entree
(10 oz) pkg Gorton's "Light
  Recipe" Fish Fillets
(9 oz) Benihana "Oriental Lite"
  Chicken in Spicy Garlic Sauce
  entree
(10 oz) Pepperidge Farm Deli
  Pastry filled w/ Turkey, Ham
  and Cheese

(9 1/4 oz) Weight Watchers Fillet of Fish au Gratin entree

(6 oz) Chun King Chicken Chow Mein

(10 oz) Le Menu "Light Style" Cheese Stuffed Shells w/ Tomato Mushroom Sauce & Broccoli entree

1 pkg Stouffer's New England Clam Chowder

(9 oz) Green Giant's Nibblers Corn on the Cob without added sauce

(10 oz) Bird's Eye Cut Green Beans

1/2 lb Ground Chuck or Ground Round

*(6 oz) Orange Juice

*(16 oz) pkg Bird's Eye Vegetable Mixture of Green Beans, Corn, Carrots and Onions

BOTTLED/CANNED

28 oz Hunt's All Natural Hickory Barbeque Sauce

8 oz Kraft Tartar Sauce

12 oz Picante Sauce/Salsa

14 oz Aunt Millie's Spaghetti Sauce w/Sweet Peppers & Italian Sausage

12 oz Chili Sauce

14 oz Heinz Lite Tomato Catsup

9 oz Mustard/Horseradish

8 oz Kraft Lite Miracle Whip Salad drsg

8 oz each Wish-Bone Lite Russian, French and Creamy Cucumber Salad drsg

8 oz Featherweight Calorie Reduced Jelly (any flavor)

10 oz Smucker's Fruit Spread (any flavor)

8 1/2 oz unswt Apricots

8 1/4 oz each Libby's Lite Pineapple Chunks and Peaches

32 fl oz Ocean Spray Low-Calorie Cranberry Juice Cocktail

6 fl oz No Salt Added V-8 Juice

15 oz Chef Boy-Ar-Dee's Beef Chili w/ Beans

6 1/2 oz Chicken of the Sea Low-Sodium White Chunk Tuna in Water

14 oz LaChoy Fancy Chinese Mixed Vegetables

*8 oz Henri's Sweet 'N Tart Salad Dressing

*6 Pak (24 oz) Mott's Natural Style Applesauce

*3 1/2 oz BACO's (Imitation Bacon Bits)

*8 1/2 oz unswt Plums

*16 oz unswt Apricots, Pineapple and Peaches

*16 oz Bush's Best Light Red Kidney Beans

BAKERY/DELI

1 Kaiser Roll

1 Seeded Hamburger Bun

1 Loaf Dark Rye/Pumpernickel Bread

2 oz FF sliced Roast Beef

3 oz Fresh Cooked Shelled Shrimp

*4 oz Fresh Shelled Shrimp

6 oz pkg Louis Rich 95-98% FF Luncheon Variety meat (any variety)

STAPLES

"Free Beverages" from *The Expresslane Diet*

Sugar Substitute (Sweet 'N Low) as desired (white or brown)

Low Sodium Spices and Herbs from *The Expresslane Diet* as desired

*for men only

SHOPPING LIST

WEEK 3
(DAYS 15 - 21)

PRODUCE

2 med Apples
2 med Grapefruit
1 med Lemon
1 sm Melon (any variety)
1 med Nectarine/Peach
1 med Orange
1 sm Pineapple
1 pint Strawberries
1 pkg Alfalfa Sprouts
2 med Stalks Broccoli
1 sm Head Cabbage
1 bunch Carrots
1 sm pkg Cauliflower Pieces
1 bunch Celery
1 med Head Lettuce
2 med Green Peppers
1/2 lb Mushrooms
1 bunch Radishes
1 bunch Scallions (green onions)
10 oz pkg Spinach Greens
2 med Tomatoes
*3 apricots/1 Dried Fig
*1 med Banana
*12 Cherries

PACKAGED GOODS

(8 oz) each Dried Figs and Apple
    Rings
(15 oz) box Dried Raisins
(10 oz) General Mills Cheerios
    Cereal
(7 oz) Quaker Puffed Rice/Wheat
    Cereal
(18 oz) Quaker or General Mills
    pkgs Regular Flavored "Quick
    Cooking" Oatmeal
(8 1/2 oz) Rye Krisp Crackers
(11 1/2 oz) Nabisco Wheatsworth
    Crackers
(12 oz) Nabisco Nilla Vanilla
    Wafers

1 pkg Thomas Toast-r-Cakes
    (Bran, Blueberry or Corn)
(11 oz) Pillsbury Soft Breadsticks
(12 oz) Thomas English Muffins
(7 oz) Prince/Enriched Spaghetti
(3 1/2 oz) Carnation's
    "Spreadables" (Turkey or
    Chicken)
*(5 oz) Uncle Ben's Brown & Wild
    Rice
*(16 oz) Nabisco Almost Home
    Oatmeal Cookies
*(12 oz) Nabisco Windmill Cookies
*(5 1/4 oz) Melba Toast
*(10 oz) Nabisco Shredded Wheat
    Biscuits
*(6 oz) Seasoned Croutons
*(3 oz) Hostess Crumb Cake

DAIRY

12 3/4 oz Lite-Line Cheese Product
    (any flavor)
8 oz Tub/Sticks Philadelphia Light
    Cream Cheese Spread
8 oz Dannon Plain Low-Fat Yogurt
1 lb Tub/Sticks Fleischmann's Diet
    Margarine
1 quart Skim Milk

FROZEN FOODS

(10 oz) Le Menu Turkey Divan
    "Light Style" entree
(11 oz) Armour Turkey Parmesan
    Classic Lite entree
(8 5/8 oz) Stouffer's Lean Cuisine
    Oriental Beef w/ Vegetables
    and Rice entree
(9 5/8 oz) Stouffer's Lean Cuisine
    Beef and Pork Cannelloni w/
    Mornay Sauce entree
(11 oz) Stouffer's Lean Cuisine
    Zucchini Lasagna entree

(3 oz) Plain Chicken Breast
(10 oz) Green Giant Baked Potato
Stuffed w/ Cheese Topping
(11 1/4 oz) Van de Kamp's Beef
Enchiladas
(10 oz) Green Giant's Long Grain
White and Wild Rice
(4 oz) single serv pkg Stokely's
Mixed Vegetables
(9 oz) pkg Bird's Eye Cauliflower
(11 oz) Eggo French Toast
*(12 oz) unswt Raspberries
*1 pt Borden's Sherbet (any fruit
flavor)
*(10 oz) Le Menu Chicken
Cacciatore entree
*(14 oz) Yoplait Yogurt Bars

BOTTLED/CANNED

8 oz each Wish-Bone Lite Italian
and Sweet N' Spicy French
Style Salad drsg
8 oz Hidden Valley Lite Ranch
Style Salad drsg
8 oz Weight Watchers/Dia-Mel
Slaw drsg
8 oz Kraft Lite Miracle Whip Salad
drsg
8 oz Hellman's Lite Mayonnaise
8 oz Cheese Sauce (Cheez Whiz)
6 Pak (24 oz) Mott's Natural Style
Applesauce
8 1/2 oz each unswt Mandarin
Oranges, Peaches and Pears
6 oz can unswt Grape Juice
15 oz Libby's Lite Pineapple
Chunks
10 oz Smucker's Fruit Spread (any
flavor)
15 oz Old El Paso Refried Beans
7 3/4 oz Featherweight Low-
Sodium Tuna or Salmon
6 oz Crabmeat or 4 1/2 oz Shrimp
16 oz Bread & Butter Pickles
14 oz LaChoy Chop Suey
Vegetables

8 1/4 oz Del Monte No Salt Added
Beets
1 can Campbell's Wonton Soup
*15 oz Green Giant's Three Bean
Salad
*3 oz Chow Mein Fried Noodles
*5 3/4 oz Lindsay Ripe Olives

BAKERY/DELI

1 French-style Roll
1 lg Hard Roll
6 oz pkg Louis Rich 95-98% FF
Luncheon Variety Meat (any
variety)
2 oz Prepared FF Turkey Breast
1 pkg "Calorie Watcher" Canadian
Style Bacon or 2 oz FF Shaved
Pork Tenderloin
*4 oz FF Shaved Pork Tenderloin

STAPLES

"Free Beverages" from *The
Expresslane Diet*
Sugar Substitute (Sweet 'N Low)
as desired (white/brown)
Low Sodium Spices and Herbs
from *The Expresslane Diet* as
desired

*for men only

Permissible Spices, Herbs, Seasonings and Condiments

Allspice
Almond Extract
Anise Seed
Baking Powder, low sodium
Baking Soda, low sodium
Basil
Bay Leaf
Bouillon Cube, low sodium
Caraway Seed
Cardamon
Catsup, low sodium
Celery Leaves, dried or fresh
Celery Seed
Chili Powder
Chives
Cinnamon
Cloves
Cocoa
Cumin Seed
Curry Powder
Dill
Fennel
Garlic, fresh or ground
Ginger, ground and root
Horseradish, roots or
  prepared low sodium
Lemon Juice/Extract
Lemon Pepper
Lime Juice/Extract
Mace
Maple, Extract or low-cal
  syrup
Marjoram
Meat Extracts, low sodium
Meat Tenderizers, low sodium
Mint

Mustard, dry, seed or
  prepared low sodium
Nutmeg
Onion, fresh, juice or powder
Orange Juice/Extract
Oregano
Paprika
Parsley, fresh or dried flakes
Peppers, fresh red or green
Pepper, black, red or white
  powder
Peppermint Extract
Pimento
Poppy Seeds
Poultry Seasoning
Rosemary
Saffron
Sage
Salt Substitute
Savory
Sesame Seeds
Sorrel
Sugar Substitute
Tarragon
Thyme
Tomato Juice, low sodium
Tumeric
Vanilla, bean or extract
Vegetable Flakes, dehydrat-
  ed without added salt
Vegetable Juice, low sodium
Vinegar, regular or herb
  flavored
Walnut Extract
Wine, Dry (1/4 cup in cooking
  per day)

Chapter 3

Expanding Your Choices: A New Exchange System

After you have completed the 21-day *Expresslane Diet*, you can continue to lose, either by electing to repeat the 21-day cycle or by designing your own menus using *The Expresslane Diet* Exchange Groups.

An "exchange group" simply means that any food in a given food group may be substituted for another. The foods in each group contain approximately the same amount of carbohydrate, protein, fat, calories and sodium. Since foods are grouped according to similar nutritional make-up, you should only exchange or substitute foods within a given group — not between groups. One selection equals one serving or one food exchange. Because many groups have sub-classifications, it's important to remember that one serving is equivalent to one choice from an entire group's list. The nine exchange groups are:

For Beginners
Frozen Classics/Convenience Entrees
Protein Pleasers
Fruits, Berries, Cherries and Much More
Vegetables Galore
Super Side Dishes
Milk Magic
Sauces Aside
Free Foods

In addition, a separate exchange system has been devised for Fast Foods that you can choose once a week.

Using the exchange lists and following a specified meal plan provides a great variety of food choices. All nutritional calculations have been done. You need only select your favorite foods from the given exchange groups. Men and women are assigned a different number of servings from each of the exchange lists. The same nutritional criteria outlined for *The Expresslane Diet* applies to foods selected from the exchange groups.

You're encouraged to spread your exchanges over three meals per day. However, if you prefer two meals or four to six, that's fine as long as you don't exceed the specified number of servings or the total amount of food for that day. Meal times can be varied to fit your schedules.

Here's a sample women's plan for *The Expresslane Diet* Exchange Groups:

BREAKFAST:

1 Fruit, Berries, Cherries and Much More
1 Milk Magic
Free Beverage

LUNCH:

2 Protein Pleasers
1 Super Side Dish
1 Vegetables Galore
1 Fruit, Berries, Cherries and Much More
Free Foods

DINNER:

1 For Beginners
1 Frozen Classic/Convenience Entree
1 Vegetables Galore
1 Sauces Aside
Free Foods

CUMULATIVE NUTRITIONAL ANALYSIS FOR EXPRESSLANE DIET
EXCHANGE GROUPS

For Beginners

Carbohydrate = 3 grams
Protein = 1 gram
Fat = 1 gram
Calories = 25
Sodium = 40 milligrams

Percent of Calories
Carbohydrate = 48%
Protein = 16%
Fat = 36%

Frozen Classics I

Carbohydrate = 32 grams
Protein = 12 grams
Fat = 4 grams
Calories = 215
Sodium = 818 milligrams

Percent of Calories
Carbohydrate = 60%
Protein = 22%
Fat = 18%

Frozen Classics II

Carbohydrate = 37 grams
Protein = 19 grams
Fat = 8 grams
Calories = 215
Sodium = 834 milligrams

Percent of Calories
Carbohydrate = 50%
Protein = 26%
Fat = 24%

Protein Pleasers

Carbohydrate = 1 gram
Protein = 7 grams
Fat = 8 grams
Calories = 108
Sodium = 214 milligrams

Percent of Calories
Carbohydrate = 4%
Protein = 27%
Fat = 69%

Fruits, Berries, Cherries and Much More

Carbohydrate = 14 grams
Protein = 0 grams
Fat = 0 grams
Calories = 56
Sodium = 23 milligrams

Percent of Calories
Carbohydrate = 100%
Protein = 0%
Fat = 0%

Vegetables Galore

Carbohydrate = 5 grams
Protein = 1 gram
Fat = 0 grams
Calories = 24
Sodium = 30 milligrams

Percent of Calories
Carbohydrate = 83%
Protein = 17%
Fat = 0%

Super Side Dishes

Carbohydrate = 23 grams
Protein = 4 grams
Fat = 2 grams
Calories = 134
Sodium = 169 milligrams

Percent of Calories
Carbohydrate = 73%
Protein = 13%
Fat = 14%

Milk Magic

Carbohydrate = 22 grams
Protein = 7 grams
Fat = 2 grams
Calories = 134
Sodium = 169 milligrams

Percent of Calories
Carbohydrate = 66%
Protein = 20%
Fat = 14%

Sauces Aside

Carbohydrate = 0 grams
Protein = 0 grams
Fat = 5 grams
Calories = 45
Sodium = 79 milligrams

Percent of Calories
Carbohydrate = 0%
Protein = 0%
Fat = 100%

Free Foods

Carbohydrate = 1 gram
Protein = 0 grams
Fat = 0 grams
Calories = 7
Sodium = 38 milligrams

Percent of Calories
Carbohydrate = 100%
Protein = 0%
Fat = 0%

THE EXPRESSLANE DIET EXCHANGE SYSTEM FOR WEIGHT CONTROL

WOMEN'S DIET PROGRAM

FOR BEGINNERS 1 serv.
FROZEN CLASSICS/
  CONVENIENCE
  ENTREES 1 serv.
PROTEIN PLEASERS 2 serv.
FRUITS, BERRIES, CHER-
  RIES & MUCH MORE 2
  serv.
VEGETABLES GALORE 2
  serv.
SUPER SIDE DISHES 1 serv.
MILK MAGIC 1 serv.
SAUCES ASIDE 1 serv.
FREE FOODS 2-3 serv.

MEN'S DIET PROGRAM

FOR BEGINNERS 1 serv.
FROZEN CLASSICS/
  CONVENIENCE
  ENTREES 1 serv.
PROTEIN PLEASERS 3 serv.
FRUITS, BERRIES,
  CHERRIES & MUCH
  MORE 2 serv.
VEGETABLES GALORE 2
  serv.
SUPER SIDE DISHES 1 1/2
  serv.
MILK MAGIC 2 serv.
SAUCES ASIDE 1 serv.
FREE FOODS 2-3 serv.

THE EXPRESSLANE DIET EXCHANGE SYSTEM DAILY NUTRITIONAL ANALYSIS

WOMEN'S DIET PROGRAM

Carbohydrate (grams) 127
Protein (grams) 47
Fat (grams) 34
Calories 943
Sodium (milligrams) 1,900

Percent of Total Calories
Carbohydrate 54%
Protein 20%
Fat 26%

MEN'S DIET PROGRAM

Carbohydrate (grams) 163
Protein (grams) 63
Fat (grams) 45
Calories 1,252
Sodium (milligrams) 2,360

Percent of Total Calories
Carbohydrate 52%
Protein 20%
Fat 28%

FOR BEGINNERS EXCHANGE GROUP

CATEGORIES:

BEVERAGES
SOUPS/CONSOMME
TOPPINGS/MIXERS

BEVERAGES:

1/4 cup unsweetened Carrot Juice
1/2 cup Ocean Spray Low Calorie Cranberry Juice Cocktail
1/2 cup Ocean Spray Low Calorie Cranberry Juice Drink
1/2 cup Hunt's No Salt Added Tomato Juice
1/2 cup Nutradiet Tomato Juice
1/2 cup Nutradiet Low Sodium Vegetable Juice Cocktail

SOUPS/CONSOMME:

ESTEE Corporation "Dietetic Soup Mixes" (as prepared)
1/2 cup Beef Vegetable Soup
1/2 cup Chicken Noodle Soup
1/2 cup Manhattan Clam Chowder
1/2 cup Mushroom Soup
1/2 cup Tomato Soup

WEIGHT WATCHERS
1 teaspoon Instant Chicken or Beef Low Sodium Bouillon
1/2 cup Low Sodium Chicken Noodle Soup (as prepared)
1/2 cup Low Sodium Tomato Soup (as prepared)

MANISCHEWITZ
1 cup Low Calorie Beet Borscht

TOPPINGS/MIXERS:
2 teaspoons BAC*Os (General Mills, Inc.)
1 tablespoon Carnation Coffee Mate

FROZEN CLASSICS/CONVENIENCE ENTREES EXCHANGE GROUP

CATEGORIES:

FROZEN CLASSICS/CONVENIENCE ENTREES I
FROZEN CLASSICS/CONVENIENCE ENTREES II
   (Subtract an additional "Sauces Aside" exchange for
   each selection from group II.)

FROZEN CLASSICS/CONVENIENCE ENTREES I:

"ARMOUR CLASSIC LITES"
1 (10 oz.) Pepper Beef Steak entree
1 (10 1/2 oz.) Chicken Chow Mein entree
1 (10 oz.) Chicken Oriental entree
1 (11 oz.) Medallions of Chicken Breast Marsala entree
1 (11 oz.) Sweet and Sour Chicken entree
1 (10 oz.) Turk and Surf entree
1 (11 oz.) Turkey Parmesan entree

"ARMOUR DINNER CLASSICS"
1 (10 1/2 oz.) Teriyaki Chicken entree

BANQUET (ConAgra Frozen Foods Company)
1 (8 oz.) Mostaccioli and Meat Sauce entree

"BANQUET'S GOURMET ENTREES"
1 (10 oz.) Chicken Cacciatore entree
1 (10 oz.) French Chicken entree
1 (10 oz.) Turkey Tetrazzini entree

"BENIHANA ORIENTAL LITES" (Benihana Frozen Foods
   Corporation)
1 (8 1/2 oz.) Glazed Chicken entree
1 (9 oz.) Shrimp and Cashews with Rice entree

CAMPBELL SOUP COMPANY'S "LE MENU LIGHT STYLE"
1 (10 oz.) Glazed Chicken Breast Dinner entree
1 (10 oz.) Chicken Cacciatore Dinner entree

HEALTHY CHOICE DINNERS

1 (8 1/2 oz.) Beef Julienne entree
1 (9 oz.) Beef Stroganoff entree
1 (8 oz.) Chicken Parmigiana entree
1 (8 oz.) Glazed Chicken entree
1 (10 oz.) Shrimp Creole entree
1 (8 oz.) Sliced Turkey entree

CONTADINA (Calreco, Inc.) "Pizzeria Kits"
  (as prepared) 1/4 Thin Crust Cheese Pizza

DINING LITE (Blue Star Foods, Inc.)
1 (8 5/8 oz.) Beef Teriyaki entree
1 (9 oz.) Carne Picado entree
1 (9 oz.) Cheese Cannelloni with Tomato Sauce entree
1 (8 1/2 oz.) Chicken Aloha — Chicken and Sauce entree
1 (11 oz.) Seafood Vegetable Medley with Rice entree
1 (10 oz.) Shrimp Creole with Rice entree

FRANCO-AMERICAN (Campbell Soup Company)
1 (7 1/2 oz.) Beef Ravioli in Meat Sauce
1 (7 1/2 oz.) Beef Ravioli Os in Meat Sauce

GREEN GIANT (Van de Kamp's Frozen Foods)
1 (9 oz.) Chicken Chow Mein entree
1 (9 oz.) Shrimp Creole with Rice entree

HORMEL (George A. Hormel and Company)
1 Cheese Burrito
1 Chicken and Rice Burrito
1 Hot Chili Burrito

KRAFT (Kraft, Incorporated)
3/4 cup Egg Noodle Dinner with Chicken (as prepared)
3/4 cup Deluxe Macaroni and Cheese Dinner (as prepared)

MORTON (ConAgra Frozen Foods Company) "LIGHT DINNERS"
1 (11 oz.) Boneless Chicken Dinner entree
1 (11 oz.) Chicken Chow Mein Dinner entree
1 (11 oz.) Sliced Beef Dinner entree

MORTON (ConAgra Frozen Foods Company) "LIGHT ENTREES"
1 (8 oz.) Chicken Chow Mein entree
1 (8 oz.) Meat Sauce and Spaghetti entree

MRS. PAUL'S (Campbell Soup Company) "
    LIGHT SEAFOOD ENTREES"
1 (11 oz.) Scallops Mediterranean entree
1 (8 1/2 oz.) Seafood Newburg entree

STOUFFER'S LEAN CUISINE (Stouffer Foods Corporation)
1 (8 oz.) Chicken a l'Orange with Almond Rice entree
1 (12 3/4 oz.) Chicken and Vegetables with Vermicelli entree
1 (11 1/4 oz.) Chicken Chow Mein with Rice entree
1 (12 3/8 oz.) Fillet of Fish Divan entree
1 (8 1/2 oz.) Glazed Chicken with Vegetable Rice entree
1 (9 5/8 oz.) Linguini with Clam Sauce entree
1 (8 5/8 oz.) Oriental Beef with Vegetables and Rice entree
1 (11 oz.) Oriental Scallops with Vegetables and Rice entree
1 (9 3/4 oz.) Tuna Lasagna with Spinach Noodles and
    Vegetables entree
1 (11 oz.) Zucchini Lasagna entree

TYSON (Tyson Foods, Incorporated)
1 (10 1/4 oz.) Chicken Oriental entree

WEIGHT WATCHERS (Foodways National, Incorporated)
1 (9 1/4 oz.) Fillet of Fish Au Gratin entree
1 (9 1/4 oz.) Imperial Chicken entree
1 (10 3/16 oz.) Sweet 'n Sour Chicken Tenders entree

FROZEN CLASSICS/CONVENIENCE ENTREES II:

- Subtract an additional "Sauces Aside" exchange for each
  selection from this list

"ARMOUR CLASSIC LITES"
1 (10 oz.) Steak Diane Mignonettes entree
1 (12 oz.) Stuffed Cabbage entree
1 (10 oz.) Szechuan Beef entree

"ARMOUR DINNER CLASSICS"
1 (11 oz.) Sirloin Roast entree

BANQUET (ConAgra Frozen Foods Company)
1 (8 oz.) Lasagna with Meat Sauce entree

"BANQUET'S GOURMET ENTREES"
1 (10 oz.) Green Pepper Steak entree
1 (10 oz.) Pasta Shells and Sauce entree
1 (10 oz.) Sliced Beef and Vegetables entree

"BENIHANA ORIENTAL LITES" (Benihana Frozen Foods
    Corporation)
1 (9 oz.) Beef and Mushrooms in Sauce with Rice and Vegetables
    entree
1 (9 oz.) Chicken in Spicy Garlic Sauce entree

THE BUDGET GOURMET'S "SLIM LINE"
1 Lasagna with Meat Sauce entree
1 Oriental Beef entree

CAMPBELL SOUP COMPANY'S "LE MENU LIGHT STYLE"
1 (10 oz.) Cheese Stuffed Shells Dinner entree
1 (10 oz.) Turkey Divan Dinner entree

CHEF BOY-AR-DEE (American Home Foods)
1/4 of 23 7/8 oz. Dinner Lasagna entree
1/4 of 21 1/4 oz. Dinner Spaghetti and Meatballs entree
1/4 of 16 7/8 oz. Hamburger Pizza (Pizza Mix as prepared)

CONTADINA (Calreco, Inc.) "Pizzeria Kits"
    (as prepared) 1/4 Thick Crust Cheese Pizza

DINING LITE (Blue Star Foods, Inc.)
1 (11 oz.) Cheese Vegetable Lasagna entree
1 (9 1/2 oz.) Chicken a la King with Rice entree
1 (11 oz.) Chicken Cacciatore with Vermicelli entree
1 (12 3/4 oz.) Chicken Vegetable Medley with Rice entree
1 (9 oz.) Veal and Vegetable Cannelloni entree
1 (11 oz.) Zucchini Lasagna

GREEN GIANT (Van de Kamp's Frozen Foods)
1 (10 oz.) Shrimp Fried Rice entree

KRAFT (Kraft, Incorporated)
1 cup American Style Spaghetti Dinner (as prepared)
1 cup Tangy Italian Style Spaghetti (as prepared)

MORTON (ConAgra Frozen Foods Company) *"LIGHT DINNERS"*
1 (11 oz.) Italian Style Ziti Dinner entree
1 (11 oz.) Turkey Tetrazzini Dinner entree

MORTON'S "LIGHT ENTREES"
1 (8 oz.) Gravy and Sliced Beef entree

MRS. PAUL'S "LIGHT SEAFOOD ENTREES" (Campbell Soup
    Company)
1 (11 oz.) Shrimp Oriental entree
1 (11 oz.) Shrimp Primavera entree

STOUFFER'S LEAN CUISINE (Stouffer Foods Corporation)
1 (11 1/2 oz.) Spaghetti with Beef and Mushroom Sauce entree
1 (10 1/4 oz.) Veal Lasagna entree

SWANSON (Campbell Soup Company) *"MAIN COURSE
    ENTREES"*
1 (9 1/4 oz.) Turkey with Gravy entree

TOMBSTONE (Tombstone Pizza)
1/4 of 22 oz. Canadian Bacon Pizza
1/4 of 20 oz. Cheese Pizza

TYSON (Tyson Foods, Incorporated)
1 (9 1/2 oz.) Chicken a l'Orange entree

WEIGHT WATCHERS (Foodways National, Incorporated)
1 (10 1/2 oz.) Chicken Cacciatore entree
1 (10 1/2 oz.) Spaghetti with Meat Sauce entree
1 (11 1/4 oz.) Ziti Macaroni entree

PROTEIN PLEASERS
EXCHANGE GROUP

CATEGORIES:

CHEESES AND SPREADS
READY TO EAT PROTEIN PLEASERS

CHEESES AND SPREADS EXCHANGES:

BORDEN
3 slices (2 oz.) Lite-Line Processed Cheese Product (any flavor
    variety)

CARNATION (Calreco, Incorporated)
1/4 container "The Spreadables" Chicken or Turkey Salad
    Sandwich Spread

DORMAN'S (N. Dorman and Company Incorporated)
1 1/4 oz. Chedda-DeLite cheese
1 1/4 oz. Chedda-Jack cheese
1 1/2 oz. Lo-Chol Imitation cheese
1 1/2 oz. Low-Sodium Mozzarella cheese
1 1/2 oz. Part Skim Mozzarella cheese
1 oz. Low-Sodium Muenster cheese
1 1/4 oz. Slim Jack cheese
1 oz. No Salt Added Swiss cheese

FRIGO
2 oz. Frigo Ricotta Cheese with part skim milk base

KRAFT (Kraft, Incorporated)
3/4 oz. Italian Blend Parmesan or Romano Grated cheese
1 oz. Brick cheese
1 oz. Caraway cheese
1 oz. Cheddar cheese
1 oz. Colby cheese
1 oz. Gouda cheese
1 oz. Monterey Jack (all varieties) cheese
1 1/2 oz. Mozzarella, low moisture part skim milk (all varieties) cheese
1 oz. Muenster cheese
1 1/2 oz. Neufchatel cheese
1 oz. Provolone cheese
1 1/2 oz. low Moisture Part Skim Scamorze cheese
1 oz. Swiss cheese
1 oz. Shredded Taco cheese
1 1/2 oz. Spreads: Pimento, Pineapple, Relish

KRAFT CASINO (Kraft, Inc.)
1 oz. Havarti cheese
1 1/4 oz. Low Moisture Mozzarella cheese
1 oz. Romano, Natural cheese

KRAFT CRACKER BARREL
1 1/4 oz. Cold Pack Cheese Food (all flavor varieties)

KRAFT GOLDEN IMAGE "Imitation Cheeses"
1 oz. Natural Cheddar cheese
1 oz. Natural Colby cheese

KRAFT MOHAWK VALLEY
1 1/4 oz. Limburger, little Gem Size Natural cheese

LAND O' LAKES (Land O' Lakes Incorporated)
1 oz. cheese, natural, except part skim
1 1/2 oz. Mozzarella cheese, part skim

SARGENTO (Sargento Cheese Company, Incorporated)
1 oz. Brick cheese
1 oz. Brie cheese
1 1/4 oz. Camembert cheese
1 oz. Colby cheese
1 oz. Colby Jack cheese
1 oz. Edam cheese
1 oz. Farmers cheese
1 oz. Finland Swiss cheese
1 oz. Gouda cheese
1 oz. Gruyere cheese
1 oz. Monterey Jack cheese
1 1/2 oz. Low Moisture part skim Mozzarella cheese
1 oz. Muenster, Red Rind cheese
1 oz. Jarlsberg cheese
1 oz. Port Wine Nut Logs
1 oz. Sharp Cheddar Nut Logs
4 oz. Pot cheese
1 oz. Provolone cheese
1 oz. Queso Blanco cheese
1 oz. Queso de Papa cheese
4 oz. Part Skim Ricotta cheese
1 1/2 oz. String cheese
1 oz. Swiss cheese
1 oz. Taco cheese
1 oz. Tilsiter cheese
1 oz. Tybo, Red Wax cheese

WEIGHT WATCHERS (Nutrition Industries Corporation)
1 1/2 oz. Natural part-skim cheese
2 oz. processed cheese product, low-sodium singles (any flavor
    variety)

READY TO EAT PROTEIN PLEASERS
(prepared without added fat):

CATEGORIES:
BEEF
FISH
LAMB
PORK
POULTRY
VEAL
OTHERS

BEEF PROTEIN PLEASERS:
(All portions 1 1/2-oz. cooked weight with all visible fat removed)
Beef Stew
Beef Tenderloin
Chuck Roast
Flank Steak
Ground Round
Ground Sirloin

AVOID:
Chipped Beef
Corned Beef
Meat Loaf
Ribs
Rump or Chuck Roast
Porterhouse Steak
T-Bone Steak
Strip Steak
Beef Tongue

FISH PROTEIN PLEASERS:
(Fresh or Frozen — All 2-oz. cooked weight portions)
Bass
Catfish
Cod
Crab
Flounder
Haddock
Halibut
Lobster

Perch
Red Snapper
Salmon
Scrod
Shrimp
Smelts
Sole
Turbot
Whitefish

FISH — CANNED:

Recommended brands include Chicken of the Sea and
    Featherweight)
4 oz. low-sodium Tuna canned in water
3 oz. low-sodium Salmon
3 medium Sardines
8 medium Oysters

AVOID:

Regular canned Clams, Crab, Lobster, Scallops or Shrimp
Regular canned Salmon or Tuna
Dried Cod
Herring, uncreamed or smoked

LAMB PROTEIN PLEASERS:

(All portions 1 1/2-oz. cooked weight with all visible fat
    removed)
Lamb Cubes
Lamb Steak
Leg of Lamb, Roast or Chop

AVOID:

Crown Roasts
Ground Lamb Patty
Lamb Chops

PORK PROTEIN PLEASERS:

(All portions 1 1/2-oz. cooked weight with all visible fat removed)
Boston Butt Steak
Ground Pork
Fresh Ham
Pork Chop or Cutlet
Pork Tenderloin Roast

AVOID:
Canadian Bacon
Ham, canned, cured, boiled or chipped
Pork Sausages, Patties or Links
Pork Spareribs
Smoked Ham Hocks or Bones

POULTRY PROTEIN PLEASERS:

(All portions 1 1/2-oz. cooked weight with all skin and visible fat
    removed)
Chicken
Turkey
Cornish Hens

AVOID:
Domestic Duck
Domestic Goose
Regular Turkey Ham Luncheon Meat

VEAL PROTEIN PLEASERS:

(All portions 1 1/2-oz. cooked weight with all visible fat removed)
Ground or Cubed Veal Steak
Veal Cutlet or Chop
Veal Riblets or Shank
Veal Roast

AVOID:
Veal Breast

OTHER PROTEIN PLEASERS:

3 slices, Butterball, Louis Rich and Oscar Mayer 95% to 98% fat
    free lunch meats (any variety)
1 Tyson's Chicken Breast Original (prepared without added fat)

FRUITS, BERRIES, CHERRIES AND MUCH MORE EXCHANGE GROUP

CATEGORIES:

CANNED CONVENIENCE
DRIED FRUITS
GARDEN FRESH
FROZEN FRUITS
FRUIT JUICES
NOVELTY FRUIT SNACKS

CANNED CONVENIENCE CHOICES:.

(1/2 cup any brand, any variety canned unsweetened fruit, drained, or fruit sauce)
Recommended brands include Del Monte Lite and Libby's Lite Canned Fruits

Examples include:
Apple or Cranberry Sauce, canned unsweetened Apricots, Cherries, Fruit Cocktail, Grapefruit, Mandarin Oranges, Peaches, Pears and Pineapple

DRIED CHOICES:

(Recommended brands include Sunmaid and Weight Watchers)
4 Apple Rings
7 Apricot Halves
2 1/2 medium Dates
1 1/2 medium Figs
2 Peach Halves
2 Pear Halves
3 medium Prunes
2 tablespoons Raisins

GARDEN FRESH FRUIT CHOICES:

1 small Apple
4 medium Apricots
1/2 medium Banana
3/4 cup Blackberries, Blueberries, Boysenberries, Loganberries, Mulberries
1 cup Raspberries
1 1/4 cup Strawberries
12 Sweet, Bing or Royal Ann Cherries
1/2 medium Grapefruit

15 small Seedless Grapes (green or red variety)
1 medium Nectarine
1 medium Orange
1 cup Papaya
1 medium Peach
1 small Pear
2 medium Persimmons
3/4 cup Pineapple
2 medium Plums
1/2 Pomegranate
2 cups Rhubarb
2 medium Tangerines

FROZEN FRUIT CHOICES:

(All selections are unsweetened)
3/4 cup Blackberries, Blueberries, Boysenberries,
    Loganberries, Mulberries
3 1/2 oz. Cranberries
1 cup Raspberries
1 1/4 cup Strawberries
1 cup Cantaloupe or Honeydew Melon
2 cups Rhubarb

FRUIT JUICE BEVERAGE CHOICES:

(All selections are unsweetened)
1/2 cup Apple Juice
3 fluid oz. Apricot Nectar
1/2 cup Grapefruit Juice
1/3 cup Grape Juice
1/2 cup Orange Juice
3 fluid oz. Peach Nectar
3 fluid oz. Pear Nectar
1/2 cup Pineapple Juice

NOVELTY FRUIT SNACK CHOICES:

1 1/2 (2.6 fluid oz.) frozen sugar-free Popsicle Ice Pops (all flavors)
1 (1 3/4 fluid oz.) frozen Blue Bunny Citrus Stick
1 (2 fluid oz.) frozen Chiquita Fruit and Juice Pop (all varieties)
1 slice (3.2 fluid oz.) frozen Good Humor Calorie-Control
    Vanilla Slice
1/4 cup frozen Haagen-Dazs Fruit Ice (all varieties)
1 (2 1/4 fluid oz.) frozen Minute Maid Fruit Juices (all flavors)
1 (3.4 fluid oz.) frozen Weight Watchers Quenchers (all flavors)

1 (3/4 fluid oz.) frozen Lifesaver Flavor Pop (all flavors)
2 frozen JELL-O Gelatin Pops (any flavor)
1 frozen JELL-O Fruit Bar (Strawberry or Mixed Berry Flavors)
2/3 Flavor Tree Fruit Roll-Up (all varieties)
1 Fruit Corners Fruit Roll-Up (all varieties)
3/4 oz. Sunmaid Dried Apple Chunks, Fruit Bits or Dried Fruit Mix

VEGETABLES GALORE
EXCHANGE GROUP

CATEGORIES:

FRESH
FROZEN
CANNED
GARNISHES

FRESH VEGETABLES GALORE:

(Unless otherwise specified, portions are 1 cup raw or 1/2 cup
     cooked — no fats added)
* = Vegetables containing 2 grams or more of dietary fiber per
     serving

Artichoke, 1 medium base and soft leaf ends
Asparagus
Bamboo Shoots
*Beans; Green, Wax or Italian
*Bean Sprouts; Mung or Soy
*Beets, 2 medium raw or 1/2 cup cooked (sliced or diced)
*Broccoli, 1 medium raw stalk or 1/2 cup cooked cuts
*Brussel Sprouts
*Cabbage
*Carrots, 1 medium raw or 1/2 cup cooked
*Cauliflower
*Collards
Eggplant
Kohlrabi
Leeks, 2 medium raw or 1/2 cup cooked
*Mushrooms
*Okra, 7 fresh pods or 1/2 cup cooked
Pea Pods or Snow Peas
Rhutabaga
*Spinach
*Tomato, 1 small raw or 1/2 cup cooked

*Turnip Greens
Water Chestnuts
*Zucchini

FROZEN VEGETABLES GALORE:

— Any fresh frozen vegetable variety without added sugar, sauces, butter or salt is permitted.
— Serving sizes are equivalent to cooked fresh vegetables listed under category I (1/2 cup cooked unless otherwise specified).
— Plain mixed frozen vegetable medleys are also limited to 1/2 cup serving, with the exception of mixtures including lentils, lima beans, peas, corn and/or potatoes, which are found in the "Super Side Dish" exchange group.
— Stokely's Single Serving Frozen Vegetables and Bird's Eye products are highly recommended.

CANNED VEGETABLES GALORE:

— Purchase any brand-name canned vegetable without added salt or sugar.
— Suggested brand names include Del Monte No Salt Added, Hunt's No Salt Added and Featherweight products.
— Serving sizes are 1/2 cup for all canned vegetables with the exception of baked beans, corn, lentils, lima beans, peas and potatoes, which are found in the "Super Side Dish" exchange group.

VEGETABLE GARNISHES GALORE:

(Dieters are permitted 1 cup of any of the following raw vegetables, separate or mixed, at lunch and dinner meals)
* = Vegetables containing 2 grams or more of dietary fiber per serving

Alfalfa Sprouts
*Celery
Chicory
*Cucumber
Endive
Escarole
Fennel
Lettuce (all varieties).
Parsley
Peppers; red, green or hot
Radishes
Scallions (green onions)
Watercress

SUPER SIDE DISH EXCHANGE GROUP

CATEGORIES:

BEANS, CORN AND MORE
BREADS AND CRACKERS
CEREALS — HOT AND COLD
PASTA, POTATOES, RICE AND STUFFING
SNACK-TYPE FOODS AND MUNCHIES
SUPER SOUPS WITHOUT A LOT OF SODIUM

* = Foods containing 2 or more grams of dietary fiber per serving

BEANS, CORN AND MORE:

*1/2 cup Campbell's Pork and Beans in Tomato Sauce
*1/2 cup Dennison's Lima Beans with Ham
*1/2 cup Health Valley Boston Baked Beans
*1/2 cup Heinz Pork 'n Beans
*1/2 cup Hormel Beans and Bacon
*1 1/2 ears frozen Bird's Eye Little Ears of Corn
*1 1/2 ears frozen Green Giant Niblet Corn on the Cob
*2/3 cup Stokely's frozen Cut Corn Kernels
*1/2 cup Health Valley Chili Con Carne

GENERIC BRAND INFORMATION:
*1/3 cup Baked Bean, No Pork
*1 1/2 Cobs of Sweet Corn
*1/2 cup Dried Peas and Beans (includes kidney, white, split,
    pinto, navy, soy and blackeye)
*1/2 cup Cooked Lentils
*3/4 cup Lima Beans (fresh or frozen)
*3/4 cup Peas (fresh, frozen or canned)
*1 cup plain cooked Pumpkin or Squash (Acorn, Butternut,
    Winter, Hubbard)

BREADS AND CRACKERS:

BREADS:
*1 Betty Crocker Muffin (1/12 pkg) (Banana, Nut, Blueberry,
    Apple or Cherry Muffin)
*1 Betty Crocker Carrot Nut or Oatmeal Raisin Muffin
*1 Dromedary (2-inch square) slice Corn Bread (from mix as
    prepared)

*1 Dromedary Corn Muffin (from mix as prepared)
*1 Flako Corn Muffin (from mix as prepared)
2 Hungry Jack Extra Rich Buttermilk Biscuits
7 Keebler Breadsticks (all varieties)
1 Pepperidge Farm Brown 'n Serve Club Roll
1 Pepperidge Farm Plain English Muffin
1 Pepperidge Farm French Style Roll
1 Pepperidge Farm Golden Twist Roll
2 Pepperidge Farm Parker House Rolls
4 Pepperidge Farm Party Rolls
1 Pepperidge Farm Sandwich Roll with Sesame Seeds
1 Pepperidge Farm Sourdough Style French Roll

GENERIC BRAND INFORMATION:
3/4 Bagel
1 1/2 Bialy
1 Biscuit (2 1/2 inches across, baking powder or refrigerator)
1 1/2 Boston Brown Bread (3 inches round by 2 inches thick)
5 slices Cocktail Rye Bread
1 1/2 Dinner Roll (2-inch roll)
3/4 English Muffin
3/4 Hamburger or Hotdog Bun
3 Pancakes (4 inches across)
3/4 Pita Pocket or Syrian Bread (6-inch width)
1 medium Plain Muffin (any variety)
1 medium Popover (2 to 3 inch)
1 1/2 slices unfrosted Raisin Bread
*1 1/2 slices Rye or Pumpernickel Bread
2 Taco Shells (6 inches across)
1 1/2 Tortilla Shells (6 inches across)
1 Waffle (4 1/2-inch square)
1 1/2 slices French, Italian, White or *Whole Wheat Bread

CRACKERS:
8 Estee Unsalted Soda Crackers
8 Featherweight Low Sodium Soda Crackers
*1 1/4 oz. Health Valley Amaranth Graham Crackers
10 Keebler Zesta Saltine Crackers
15 Manischewitz Matzo Crackers
1 oz. Manischewitz Matzo Sheets
9 Manischewitz Tam Crackers
2 (1 oz.) Nabisco Crown Pilot Crackers

40 (1 oz.) Nabisco Dandy Soup and Oyster Crackers
2 Nabisco Holland Rusks
*5 Nabisco Sesame Seed Meal Mates Wafers
36 (1 oz.) Nabisco Oysterettes Oyster Crackers
2 (1 oz.) Nabisco Royal Lunch Milk Crackers
2 (1 oz.) Nabisco Sea Rounds Crackers
11 Nabisco Sociables
*6 Nabisco Low-Salt or Original Triscuit Crackers
6 Nabisco Uneeda Biscuits, Unsalted Tops
7 Nabisco Waverly Crackers
*14 Nabisco Original, Low-Salt or Cheese Wheat Thins
4 Nabisco Zweiback Toast
7 Pepperidge Farm English Wafer Biscuits
40 Pepperidge Farm Goldfish Crackers (all varieties)
8 Pepperidge Farm Snack Sticks (all varieties)
14 Ralston Animal Crackers
10 Ralston Unsalted Tops Crackers
67 (1 oz.) Ralston Oyster Crackers
*5 Ralston Ry Krisp (triple crackers — 1 1/4 oz.) all varieties
*8 Weight Watchers Crispbreads (golden wheat, garlic or
       harvest rice)

GENERIC BRAND INFORMATION:
6 Butter-based Crackers
*5 Graham Crackers
*8 slices Melba Toast (any variety)

CEREALS — HOT AND COLD:

HOT CEREALS:
*1 packet (1 1/4 oz.) General Mills Instant Total Oatmeal
       (cooked — Apple and Cinnamon flavor)
*1 1/2 packets (1 1/2 oz.) General Mills Instant Total Oatmeal
       (cooked — Original flavor)
1 packet Nabisco Cream of Wheat Mix 'n Eat (all flavors except
       original)
3 1/2 tablespoons Quaker Enriched Corn Meal, White or Yellow
       (uncooked)
*1/3 cup Quaker Oat Bran Cereal (uncooked)
*2/3 cup Quaker cooked Quick or Old Fashioned Cereal
*1 cup Quaker Instant Oatmeal (cooked — regular flavor)
*3/4 cup Quaker Instant Apple and Cinnamon Oatmeal
       (cooked — all varieties)

*1 packet (1 1/4 oz.) Quaker Fruit and Cream Oatmeal
   (all varieties)
*1 packet (3/4 cup cooked) Quaker Real Honey
   and Graham Oatmeal

COLD CEREALS:

GENERAL MILLS
*2/3 cup Bran Muffin Crisp
*1 1/2 cup Cheerios
3/4 cup Cinnamon Toast Crunch
*3/4 cup Clusters
*1 cup Corn Total
1 cup Country Corn Flakes
*3/4 cup Crispy Wheats 'n Raisins
*1 cup Fiber One
1 cup Kaboom
1 1/2 cups Kix
3/4 cup Oatmeal Raisin Crisp
*1/2 cup Raisin Nut Bran
*1 cup Total
*1 cup Wheaties

HEALTH VALLEY
*1 oz. Health Crunch (all varieties)
*1 oz. Hearts O'Bran
*1 oz. Orangeola Cereal (all varieties)
1 1/4 oz. Puffed Corn, Rice or Wheat
*1 oz. Raisin Bran Flakes
*1 oz. Real Granola (all varieties)
*1 oz. Stoned Wheat Flakes

KELLOGG'S
*1/2 cup All Bran
*1 cup All Bran with Extra Fiber
*3/4 cup All Bran Fruit and Almonds
1 cup Apple Jacks
*1/2 cup Bran Buds
1 cup Corn Flakes
*3/4 cup Fruitful Bran
*3/4 cup Honey and Nut Corn Flakes
*3/4 cup Just Right with Fruit
1 cup Product 19
*3/4 cup Raisin Bran
*3/4 cup Raisin Squares

1 cup Rice Krispies
1 cup Special K

NABISCO
*1 1/2 oz. 100% Bran
*1 oz. Toasted Wheat and Raisins
*1 oz. Spoon Size Shredded Wheat
1 oz. Team Flakes

NUTRI GRAIN (Kellogg Company)
*1/2 cup Almond Raisin
*1/2 cup Corn
*3/4 cup Wheat
*2/3 cup Wheat and Raisins

POST
1 oz. Alpha Bits
*1 oz. Fortified Oat Flakes
*1 1/4 oz. Fruit and Fibre (all varieties)
*1 oz. Grape Nuts or Raisin Grape Nuts
*1 1/4 oz. Grape-Nut Flakes
*1 1/4 oz. Natural Bran Flakes
*1 1/2 oz. Natural Raisin Bran
1 cup Toasties Corn Flakes

QUAKER
2 1/2 cups Halfsies
1 1/2 cups King Vitamin
3/4 cup Life (regular or cinnamon)
*2/3 cup Corn Bran
2 1/2 cups Puffed Wheat or Puffed Rice
*1 1/2 Biscuits Shredded Wheat
*3/4 cup Unprocessed Bran

RALSTON
*3/4 cup Bran Chex
*1 1/4 cup Corn Chex
*3/4 cup Crispy Oatmeal and Raisin Chex
*3/4 cup Wheat Chex
*3/4 cup Wheat and Raisin Chex
1 1/4 cup Corn Flakes
1 1/4 cup Crispy Rice
*1 cup 40% Bran Flakes
*1 1/2 cups Raisin Bran
1 1/2 cup Tasteeos

PASTA, POTATOES, RICE AND STUFFING:

PASTA:
1/2 cup cooked Creamette Egg Noodles
1/2 cup cooked Creamette Macaroni, Spaghetti, miscellaneous
    Pasta products
1/2 cup Golden Grain's Noodle Roni Parmesano (as prepared)

GENERIC BRAND INFORMATION:
3/4 cup any brand cooked plain Macaroni, Noodles, Spaghetti,
    Pasta

POTATOES:
1/2 cup Betty Crocker's Chicken 'n Herb Potatoes (as prepared)
1/2 cup Betty Crocker's Hash Brown Potatoes
1/2 cup French's Creamy Italian-style Potatoes with Parmesan
    Cheese
3/4 cup French's Dinner Potato Pancakes (as prepared)
1/2 cup French's Creamy Stroganoff Potatoes (as prepared)
5 oz. Ore-Ida Cheddar Browns (as prepared)
5 oz. Ore-Ida Southern Style Hash Browns (as purchased)
4 oz. Ore-Ida Home Style Potato Wedges (as purchased)
4 1/2 oz. Ore-Ida Crinkle Cut Lites (as purchased)
6 oz. Ore-Ida Potatoes O'Brien (as purchased)

GENERIC BRAND INFORMATION:
*1 medium Potato, baked or boiled
*3/4 cup Mashed Potato (without fat added)
10 French Fried Potatoes
1/4 cup Hash Brown Potatoes

RICE:
2/3 cup Featherweight Low-Sodium Spanish Rice (cooked)
1/2 cup Golden Grain Beef Rice-A-Roni (as prepared)
1/2 cup Golden Grain Chicken Rice-A-Roni (as prepared)
1/2 cup Golden Grain Spanish Rice-A-Roni (as prepared)

GREEN GIANT'S LINE OF "RICE ORIGINALS" (as prepared):
1/2 cup Green Giant's Rice and Broccoli in Flavored Cheese Sauce
1/2 cup Green Giant's Rice Medley
1/2 cup Green Giant's Rice Pilaf
1/2 cup Green Giant's White and Wild Rice
1/2 cup La Choy Canned Fried Rice
1/2 cup Lipton Chicken Flavor Rice and Sauce Mix (as prepared)

1/2 cup Lipton Mushroom Rice and Sauce Mix (as prepared)

1/2 cup Lipton Spanish Rice and Sauce Mix (as prepared)

3/4 cup regular Minute Rice (prepared without salt or butter)

1/2 cup Minute Rice Drumstick Rice Mix (prepared without salt or butter)

1/2 cup Minute Rice Long Grain and Wild Rice Mix (prepared without salt or butter)

1/2 cup Minute Rice Rib Roast Rice Mix (prepared without salt or butter)

1/2 of 5 7/8 oz. package Stouffer's Apple Pecan Rice

1/2 of 6 oz. package Stouffer's Rice Medley

1/2 cup Uncle Ben's Brown and Wild Rice (prepared without salt or butter)

2/3 cup Uncle Ben's Converted Brand Rice (prepared without salt or butter)

1/2 cup Uncle Ben's Fast-Cooking Long Grain and Wild Rice (prepared without butter)

2/3 cup Uncle Ben's Select Brown Rice (prepared without salt or butter)

1/2 cup Country Inn Broccoli Rice Au Gratin (prepared without butter)

1/2 cup Country Inn Rice Florentine (prepared without butter)

1/2 cup Country Inn Rice Oriental with Vegetables (prepared without butter)

1/2 cup Country Inn Vegetable Rice Medley (prepared without butter)

GENERIC BRAND INFORMATION:

1/2 cup any brand cooked plain rice: brown, regular, wild or instant prepared without added fats or salt

*3/4 cup cooked any brand plain Barley or Buckwheat

STUFFING:

"STOVE TOP STUFFING MIXES"

1 serving as packaged:

American New England Stuffing Mix

Americana San Francisco Stuffing Mix

Beef Stuffing Mix

Chicken Flavor Stuffing Mix

Cornbread Stuffing Mix

Long Grain & Wild Rice Stuffing Mix

Pork Stuffing Mix

Savory Herbs Stuffing Mix
Turkey Stuffing Mix
Wild Rice Stuffing Mix
1/2 cup Uncle Ben's Instant Stuffing Mix (prepared without butter)

GENERIC BRAND INFORMATION:
4 tablespoons Cornmeal or Matzo Meal (dry)
1/4 cup prepared bread stuffing (without added salt or butter)

SNACK-TYPE FOODS AND MUNCHIES:

3 Chico San Cakes (any variety)
25 Estee Unsalted Pretzel Rods
18 Featherweight Low-Sodium Pretzel Rods
1 oz. Rold Gold Pretzel Rods
1 oz. Rold Gold Pretzel Sticks
1 oz. Rold Gold Pretzel Twists
1 oz. Health Valley Pretzels
1 oz. Health Valley Low-Sodium Pretzels

"MR. SALTY" BRAND
2 (1 oz.) Dutch Pretzels
29 (1 oz.) Pretzel Juniors, plain or butter flavor
10 (1 oz.) Pretzel Logs
16 (1 oz.) Pretzel Minis
22 (1 oz.) Pretzel Nuggets
24 (1 oz.) Pretzel Rings, plain or butter flavor
2 (1 oz.) Pretzel Rods
5 (1 oz.) Pretzel Twists, plain or butter flavor
45 (1 oz.) Veri-Thin Pretzel Sticks

"SKINNY MUNCHIES" BRAND
1 oz. (2 packages) Nacho Cheese
1 oz. (2 packages) Smoky Bar-B-Que
1 oz. (2 packages) Toasted Onion

SUPER SOUPS WITHOUT A LOT OF SODIUM:

CAMPBELL'S — "Ready to Serve Low-Sodium" Line of Soups
1 cup Chicken with Noodles
2/3 cup Chunky Beef and Mushroom
*2/3 cup Split Pea
*1 cup Tomato with Tomato Pieces

FEATHERWEIGHT — "Ready to Serve Low-Sodium" Line of
   Soups
2 cups Chicken Noodle
2 cups Tomato

HEALTH VALLEY — "Ready to Serve Soups"
*1/2 cup Bean
1 cup Tomato
*1 cup Chunky Minestrone
*1 cup Chunky Split Pea
*1 cup Chunky Vegetable

MILK MAGIC EXCHANGE GROUP

CATEGORIES:

BEVY OF BEVERAGES
FROZEN DAIRY DELIGHTS
PUDDINGS AND MOUSSE
YOGURT

BEVY OF BEVERAGES:

2 packages Alba Fit 'N Frosty Beverages (all flavors)
2 packages Alba Hot Cocoa
2 envelopes Carnation Hot Cocoa Mixes 70 Calorie Beverage
6 fluid oz. Dannon Dan'Up Yogurt Drink (Strawberry flavor)
6 fluid oz. Dean's Yogurt To Go Drink (all flavors)
1 tablespoon Nestle Quik Chocolate or Strawberry Flavor Mix
24 fluid oz. Weight Watchers Chocolate Fudge Shake
24 fluid oz. Weight Watchers Orange Sherbet Shake
14 fluid oz. Weight Watchers Chocolate or Chocolate
   Marshmallow Hot Cocoa

GENERIC BRANDS BEVERAGES:
1 1/2 cups (12 fluid oz.) Skim Milk
1 1/4 cups (10 fluid oz.) 1% Milk or Buttermilk made from
   Skim Milk
1 cup (8 fluid oz.) 2% Milk
1/3 cup Powdered Non-Fat Dry Milk
6 fluid oz. Canned Evaporated Skim Milk

FROZEN DAIRY DELIGHTS:

1/2 cup Blue Bunny Ice Milk (vanilla flavor)
1/2 cup Blue Bunny Sherbet (any flavor)
1 (2 1/2 fluid oz.) Blue Bunny Sherbet Push-up (any flavor)
1/2 cup Borden's Ice Milk (any flavor)
2/3 cup Breyer's Natural Light Ice Cream (any flavor without nuts)
2 Creamsicle Cream Pops (any flavor)
1 cup (8 fluid oz.) Danny in a Cup frozen Chocolate or Vanilla Yogurt
2 slices (6.4 fluid oz.) Good Humor Calorie-Control Vanilla Slices
2/3 cup Hi-Lite Ice Milk (chocolate or vanilla)
1 1/2 JELL-O Pudding Pop (all flavors except chocolate covered)
2/3 cup Kemp's Ice Milk (all flavors)
1/2 cup Kemp's Sherbet (all flavors)
2/3 cup Land O' Lakes Ice Milk (all varieties)
1/2 cup Land O' Lakes Sherbet (all fruit flavors)
1/2 cup Sealtest low fat (98% fat free) frozen Strawberry Yogurt
1/2 cup Sealtest Light 'n Lively Ice Milk (any flavor)
2/3 cup Weight Watchers Frozen Dietary Dessert (all flavors)
1 (2.75 fluid oz.) Weight Watchers Vanilla Ice Cream Sandwich Bar
2 bars (3.5 oz.) Weight Watchers Orange Vanilla Treat
1/2 cup Yoplait Soft Frozen Yogurt (any flavor)

PUDDINGS AND MOUSSE:

1 cup Estee Dietetic Pudding (all varieties as prepared)
2/3 cup Featherweight Calorie-Reduced Chocolate Mousse Mix (as prepared)
1 cup Featherweight Low Calorie Pudding Mix (all varieties as prepared)
1/2 cup JELL-O Rich and Luscious Mousse (all flavors as prepared with skim milk)
1/2 cup Swiss Miss Pudding Packs (Tapioca or Vanilla)
1 cup Weight Watchers Cheesecake Mousse (as prepared)
2/3 cup Weight Watchers Pudding (Butterscotch, Chocolate or Vanilla, as prepared)

YOGURT:

1 1/2 cups (12 fluid oz.) Dannon Lite Yogurt (any flavor)
1 cup (8 fluid oz.) Dannon Plain Low-Fat Yogurt
1/2 cup (4 fluid oz.) Dannon Fruit on the Bottom Yogurt (any flavor)
1/2 cup (4 fluid oz.) Dannon Hearty Nuts and Raisins Yogurt

1 cup (8 fluid oz.) Gaymont French Vanilla Low-Fat Yogurt
1 1/2 cups (12 fluid oz.) Weight Watchers Plain Nonfat Yogurt
2/3 cup (6 fluid oz.) Yoplait Extra Mild Plain Yogurt

SAUCES ASIDE EXCHANGE GROUP

CATEGORIES:
MIXERS (OIL, SALAD DRESSING)
SPREADABLES (SPREADS, MARGARINE, MAYONNAISE)
NUTS, SEEDS, TOPPINGS

MIXERS:

1 teaspoon oil (Corn, Cottonseed, Olive, Peanut, Safflower,
    Soybean and Sunflower)
1 tablespoon regular salad dressing (any variety)
2 tablespoons lite or calorie-reduced salad dressing (any variety)
*Suggested brands of calorie-reduced salad dressings include:
    Featherweight
    Good Seasons
    Henri's
    Hidden Valley Ranch
    Kraft
    Seven Seas
    Weight Watchers
    Wish-Bone

SPREADABLES:

SPREADS:
1 tablespoon (1/2 oz.) Regular Cream Cheese (Soft or Whipped)
2 tablespoons (1 oz.) Lite Whipped Cream Cheese
2 teaspoons Tartar Sauce

MARGARINE:
*Purchase brands, such as Fleischmann's and Mazola, listing "
    liquid" permissible oil (from Mixers I) as first ingredients
1 tablespoon Diet or Reduced Calorie Margarine
2 teaspoons Light Spread Margarine
1 1/2 teaspoons Regular Soft Spread Margarine
1 1/2 teaspoons Regular Squeeze Margarine
1 1/2 teaspoons Regular Stick Margarine
2 teaspoons Regular Whipped Margarine

MAYONNAISE:
1 tablespoon Lite Mayonnaise
1 teaspoon Regular Mayonnaise
1 tablespoon Lite Mayonnaise Type Salad Dressing
2 teaspoons Regular Mayonnaise Type Salad Dressing

NUTS, SEEDS TOPPINGS:
* Purchased without added fat or salt
6 Whole Dry Roasted Almonds
2 Whole Brazil Nuts
4 Whole Dry Roasted Cashews
20 small/10 large Dry Roasted Peanuts
5 Pecan Halves
1 tablespoon Pine Nuts
15 Shelled Pistachios
2 teaspoons Pumpkin Seeds
1 tablespoon Sesame Seeds
1 tablespoon Sunflower Seeds
4 Walnut Halves, Black or English

SAUCES ASIDE TO AVOID:
Bacon
Imitation Bacon; limit to one teaspoon per serving
Butter; Stick or Whipped
Chicken Fat
Chitterlings, Fried
Coconut; Fresh or Dried
Coffee Creamer; Liquid or Powder
Sour Cream
Whipping Cream
Gravies
Lard
Salt Pork

FREE FOOD EXCHANGE GROUP

RULES:

— Consume as desired at meal time or snacks unless otherwise stated.
— Where quantities are indicated limit to 1 serving per day from a given category

> **CATEGORIES:**
>
> BEVERAGES
> DESSERTS
> FRUIT FLAVORED DRINKS
> JAM, JELLIES, SPREADS
> SYRUPS, SAUCES, DIPS, SALAD DRESSINGS
> MISCELLANEOUS

BEVERAGES:

(Caffeine-free beverage options are recommended)
Coffee; Hot or Cold, Regular or Decaf (all varieties without added sugar)
Tea; Hot or Cold, Regular or Decaf (all varieties without added sugar)
Water; Tap or Carbonated (plain or fruit flavored without added sugar)
Soft Drinks; Sugar-free Club Soda or Tonic and Soda (caffeine-free or regular sugar-free)

DESSERTS:

1/2 cup Dia-Mel Dietetic Gelatin (all flavors)
1/2 cup D-Zerta Low Calorie Gelatin (all flavors)
1/2 cup Estee Dietetic Gelatin (all flavors)
1/2 cup Featherweight Dietetic Gelatin (all flavors)
1/2 cup Sugar Free JELL-O Gelatin (all flavors)

FRUIT FLAVORED DRINKS:

Country Time Sugar Free Drink Mix (all flavors)
Crystal Light Sugar Free Drink Mix (all flavors)
Kool-Aid Sugar Free Soft Drink Mix (all flavors)
1 cup (8 fluid oz.) Minute Maid Crystals (all flavors Lite Mix)
Sunkist Light Sugar Free Drink (all flavors)
Tang Sugar Free Breakfast Beverage Crystals (as prepared)
6 fluid oz. Minute Maid Light and Juicy Fruit Drink (all flavors)

JAM, JELLIES, SPREADS:

1 teaspoon any variety or flavor Reduced Calorie Jam, Jelly, Preserve
— Recommended brands include: Dia-Mel, Featherweight, Kraft, Nutradiet

SYRUPS, SAUCES, DIPS, SALAD DRESSINGS:

SYRUPS:

1 tablespoon Dia-Mel Dietetic Blueberry, Chocolate or Pancake Syrup
1 tablespoon Featherweight Reduced Calorie Syrup (all flavors)
1 tablespoon Nutradiet Flavored Pancake Syrup

SAUCES:

1 tablespoon prepared Chili Sauce
Horseradish
Hot Pepper and Tobasco Sauce
1 tablespoon prepared Low-Sodium Ketchup
1 tablespoon prepared Low-Sodium Mustard
Low-Sodium Soy Sauce
Vinegar (all varieties)

DIPS:

1 tablespoon Dean's Extra Light Dips (all varieties)
1 tablespoon Land O'Lakes Lean Cream Dip (all varieties)

SALAD DRESSING:

1 tablespoon Dia-Mel Dietetic Salad Dressing (all varieties)
1 tablespoon Durkee Weight Watcher Salad Dressing Mixes (all varieties)
1 tablespoon Estee Dietetic Salad Dressing (all varieties)
1 tablespoon Featherweight Low Calorie Salad Dressing (all varieties)
1 tablespoon Good Seasons No Oil Italian Salad Dressing Mix
1 teaspoon Nutradiet Reduced Calorie Mayonnaise
1 tablespoon Weight Watchers Tomato Vinaigrette, Caesar, French Style or Italian Salad Dressing
1 teaspoon Wish-Bone Lite Salad Dressing (any variety)

MISCELLANEOUS:

2 pieces Sugar Free Hard Candy
1 tablespoon Cool Whip Non-dairy Whipped Topping
5 sticks Sugar Free Chewing Gum

Flavorings and Extracts (any)
The Juice from one Fresh Lemon or Lime
Non-stick Spray Coating
Sugar substitutes containing Saccharin, Aspartame or
    Acesulfame-K

EXCHANGING
FAST FOOD FAVORITES

Once a week, you can substitute any of the following "Fast Foods" for assigned *Expresslane Diet* Exchange Groups. Do not add any extra condiments or substitute different size entrees for those listed. Foods have been selected to meet nutritional criteria for *The Expresslane Diet*.

You'll find some of the selections can only be worked into maintenance programs because of higher fat and calorie contents. The choice is yours. Are these foods worth it to you?

FAST FOOD CHAIN LUNCH:	EXPRESSLANE DIET EXCHANGE EQUIVALENTS:
ARBY'S	
1 Regular Fish Sandwich	1 Frozen Classic/Convenience Entree I + 1 Protein Pleaser + 1 Sauces Aside + 1 Fruits, Berries, Cherries & Much More
1 French Dip Sandwich	1 Frozen Classic/Convenience Entree I + 1 Protein Pleaser + 1/2 Milk Magic + 1 Vegetable Galore
1 Junior Roast Beef Sandwich	1 Super Side Dish + 1 Protein Pleaser
1 Regular Roast Beef Sandwich	1 Frozen Classic/Convenience Entree I + 1/2 Protein Pleaser

ARTHUR TREACHERS

1 Chicken Sandwich	1 Frozen Classic/Convenience Entree I + 1 Fruits, Berries, Cherries & Much More + 1 Protein Pleaser
2 Pieces Fried Chicken	1/2 Frozen Classic/Convenience Entree I + 2 Protein Pleasers + 1/2 Fruits, Berries, Cherries & Much More
1 Regular Fish Sandwich	1 Frozen Classic/Convenience Entree II + 1/2 Fruits, Berries, Cherries & Much More + 1 1/2 Sauces Aside
2 Pieces Fried Fish	1/2 Frozen Classic/Convenience Entree I + 2 Protein Pleasers + 1/2 Fruits, Berries, Cherries & Much More

BURGER KING

1 Regular Hamburger	1 1/2 Protein Pleaser + 1 Super Side Dish + 1/4 Fruits, Berries, Cherries & Much More
1 Regular Cheeseburger	2 1/4 Protein Pleaser + 2 Fruits, Berries, Cherries & Much More
1 Whaler Sandwich	1 Frozen Classic/Convenience Entree II + 2 Protein Pleasers + 1 Sauces Aside + 1 Super Side Dish
1 Order Regular French Fries	1 Super Side Dish + 2 Sauces Aside
1 Vanilla or Chocolate Milkshake	1 Milk Magic + 1 Fruits, Berries, Cherries & Much More + 1 Super Side Dish + 1 1/2 Sauces Aside

DAIRY QUEEN

1 Regular Fish Sandwich	1 Frozen Classic/Convenience Entree I + 1 Protein Pleaser + 1/2 Fruits, Berries, Cherries & Much More

1 Regular Hamburger	1 Frozen Classic/Convenience Entree I + 1 Protein Pleaser + 1/2 Sauces Aside
1 Order Regular French Fries	1 Super Side Dish + 2 Sauces Aside
1 Small Ice Cream in Cone	1/2 Protein Pleaser + 1 Fruits, Berries, Cherries & Much More
1 Ice Cream Sandwich	1 Super Side Dish + 1/2 Sauces Aside
1 Rootbeer Float	1 Milk Magic + 2 Fruits, Berries, Cherries & Much More + 1 Sauces Aside + 1 Vegetables Galore
1 Mr. Misty Kiss	1 Fruits, Berries, Cherries & Much More
1 Small Milkshake (any flavor)	1 Milk Magic + 1 Super Side Dish + 1 1/2 Sauces Aside

HARDEE'S

1 Fisherman Fillet	1 Frozen Classic/Convenience Entree I + 1 1/2 Protein Pleaser + 1/2 Milk Magic
1 Regular Hamburger	1 Frozen Classic/Convenience Entree I + 1 Protein Pleaser
1 Mushroom 'n Swiss Hamburger	1 Frozen Classic/Convenience Entree I + 2 Protein Pleasers + 1/2 Milk Magic + 1 Vegetables Galore

JACK IN THE BOX

1 Regular Hamburger	1 Super Side Dish + 1 Vegetables Galore + 1 Protein Pleaser

KENTUCKY FRIED CHICKEN

1 Side Breast Original Recipe Chicken	1 1/2 Protein Pleaser + 1 Vegetables Galore
1 Chicken Breast Filet Sandwich	1 Frozen Classic/Convenience Entree I + 2 Protein Pleasers + 1/2 Sauces Aside

1 Order Regular French Fries	1 Super Side Dish + 1 Sauces Aside + 1/3 Fruits, Berries, Cherries & Much More
1 Order Coleslaw	1 Fruits, Berries, Cherries & Much More + 1 1/2 Sauces Aside
1 Cob of Corn	1/2 Super Side Dish + 1/2 Protein Pleaser + 1 Fruits, Berries, Cherries & Much More
1/2 cup Plain Mashed Potato	1/2 Super Side Dish
1 Plain Roll	1/2 Super Side Dish

LONG JOHN SILVER

1 Serving Clam Chowder	1/2 Super Side Dish + 1/2 Vegetables Galore + 1/2 Sauces Aside
1 Cob of Corn	1/2 Super Side Dish + 1/2 Protein Pleaser + 1 Fruits, Berries, Cherries & Much More

MCDONALD'S

1 Egg McMuffin	1 Frozen Classic/Convenience Entree I + 1 Protein Pleaser
1 Order Hot Cakes with Butter and Syrup	1 Frozen Classic/Convenience Entree I + 1 Super Side Dish + 1 Sauces Aside + 2 Fruits, Berries, Cherries & Much More
1 Chicken Salad Oriental (with 1 package Lite Vinaigrette Dressing)	1 Super Side Dish + 1/2 Sauces Aside
1 Shrimp Salad (with 1 package Lite Vinaigrette Dressing)	1 Protein Pleaser + 1/2 Sauces Aside + 1/2 Fruits, Berries, Cherries & Much More
1 Regular Hamburger	1 Frozen Classic/Convenience Entree I + 1 Sauces Aside
1 Regular Cheeseburger	1 Protein Pleaser + 1 Milk Magic + 1/2 Sauces Aside + 1/2 Fruits, Berries, Cherries & Much More

1 Filet-O-Fish Sandwich	1 Frozen Classic/Convenience Entree I + 1 Vegetables Galore + 4 Sauces Aside
1 Order 6-Piece Chicken McNuggets with 1 packet Sauce (any flavor)	2 Protein Pleaser + 1 Super Side Dish + 1 For Beginners
1 Order Regular French Fries	1 Super Side Dish + 1 Sauces Aside + 1/3 Fruits, Berries, Cherries & Much More
1 Soft Serve Ice Cream in Cone	1 Super Side Dish + 1/2 Sauces Aside + 1 Vegetables Galore
1 Milkshake (any flavor)	1 Milk Magic + 1 Super Side Dish + 1 Sauces Aside + 1 Fruits, Berries, Cherries & Much More

PIZZA HUT

1/2 (10-inch) Thin 'n Crispy Cheese Pizza	1 Frozen Classic/Convenience Entree I + 1 Protein Pleaser + 1 Fruits, Berries, Cherries & Much More
1/2 (10-inch) Thin 'n Crispy Pepperoni Pizza	1 Frozen Classic/Convenience Entree I + 1 Protein Pleaser + 1 Fruits, Berries, Cherries & Much More
1/2 (10-inch) Thin 'n Crispy Supreme Pizza	1 Frozen Classic/Convenience Entree I + 1 Protein Pleaser + 1 Sauces Aside + 1 Fruits, Berries, Cherries & Much More
1/2 (10-inch) Thick 'n Chewy Cheese Pizza	1 Frozen Classic/Convenience Entree II + 1/2 Protein Pleaser + 1/2 Super Side Dish + 1/2 Milk Magic + 1 Fruits, Berries, Cherries & Much More
1/2 (10-inch) Thick 'n Chewy Pepperoni Pizza	1 Frozen Classic/Convenience Entree I + 1 Protein Pleaser + 1 Super Side Dish + 1/2 Fruits, Berries, Cherries & Much More

1/2 (10-inch) Thick 'n Chewy Supreme Pizza	1 Frozen Classic/Convenience Entree I + 1 1/2 Protein Pleasers + 1/2 Super Side Dish + 1/4 Milk Magic + 1 Fruits, Berries, Cherries & Much More

TACO BELL

1 Bean Burrito	1 Frozen Classic/Convenience Entree I + 1 Super Side Dish + 1 Sauces Aside
1 Combination Burrito	1 Frozen Classic/Convenience Entree I + 1 Vegetables Galore + 1 1/2 Sauces Aside
1 Cheesarito	1 Frozen Classic/Convenience Entree I + 1 For Beginners + 1 1/2 Sauces Aside
1 Order Frijoles and Cheese with 1 Taco Sauce Packet	1 Frozen Classic/Convenience Entree I
1 Regular Hamburger	1 Protein Pleaser + 1 Super Side Dish
1 Seafood Salad	1 1/2 Protein Pleasers + 1/2 Milk Magic
1 Tostada	1 For Beginners + 1 Milk Magic + 1/2 Sauces Aside

WENDY'S

1 Chicken Sandwich on Multigrain Bread	1 Frozen Classic/Convenience Entree I + 1/2 Protein Pleaser
1 Order Chicken A la King	1 Frozen Classic/Convenience Entree I + 1 Super Side Dish + 1/2 Vegetables Galore
1 Regular Hamburger	3 Protein Pleasers + 1 Sauces Aside + 1/2 Fruits, Berries, Cherries & Much More
1 Regular Cheeseburger	3 1/2 Protein Pleasers + 1 Milk Magic +1 Sauces Aside + 1/2 Fruits, Berries, Cherries & Much More

1 (8.8 oz.) Plain Baked Potato	2 Super Side Dishes
1 cup (8 oz.) Chili Con Carne	1/2 Frozen Classic/Convenience Entree I + 1 Protein Pleaser + 1/2 Super Side Dish
1 Order Regular French Fries	1 Super Side Dish + 3 Sauces Aside + 1 1/4 Fruits, Berries, Cherries & Much More
1 (12 oz.) Frosty Dairy Dessert	1 Milk Magic + 1/2 Super Side Dish + 1 1/2 Fruits, Berries, Cherries & Much More + 2 Sauces Aside

Chapter 4

Understanding What's Going Down

While our strategies for losing weight have changed over the years, the "science" of losing weight has not. The simple fact remains: It takes a caloric deficit of 3,500 calories to lose one pound of body fat.

Initially, it matters not to our bodies whether this deficit results from a bizarre low-calorie candy bar diet or a nutritionally balanced diet. However, scientists have discovered that a calorie isn't a calorie isn't a calorie. Fats, which contain two and one-quarter times the calories per gram as pure proteins or carbohydrates, aren't used very well. Food is used faster and less fat is stored with a high-carbohydrate diet, such as *The Expresslane Diet.* Moreover, "yo-yo" dieters, or those persons losing and gaining the same ten pounds again and again, eventually find their metabolism has slowed down to such an extent that it's extremely difficult to lose weight even if they "starve." Their metabolisms have decreased 10 to 15 percent to compensate for periods of starvation. They have literally increased their "set point weights." What's a dieter to do?

In this era of computerization, one might liken our bodies to programmed ticker tapes — machines that automatically add up and register calorie inputs and expenditures. For example, if you decrease your typical daily calorie intake by approximately 500 calories, you should lose one pound of body fat each week. For most of us who have ever battled with a weight problem, however, instead of progressing, we seem to get stuck on "plateaus."

While we can lose weight, more often than not, we regain the original weight and add a few pounds. Then we lose weight again and gain everything back again. In fact, nine out of ten dieters are unsuccessful. Some people only change their eating habits for short periods of time and don't get any exercise. Sensible eating habits, along with regular exercise, are the keys to successful weight control.

What's Right for You?

Prudent lifestyles can become permanent fixtures. The big mistake most dieters make is choosing diets that are simply too hard to stay on. Some menus barely stimulate a rabbit's appetite. Some require too much time selecting, preparing, weighing or measuring foods. Monitoring is another problem. At professional diet centers, the daily or weekly weigh-ins can become a grind when scheduled appointments conflict with our precious free time. On diets from Monday through Friday, weekend splurges prove disastrous, making our efforts fruitless.

Some dieters complain they find themselves becoming antisocial. They feel obligated to beg off invitations from friends and family, fearing someone will find out they are dieting. Someone may pick a place where there is absolutely nothing permissible for them to eat. Defeat, defeat, defeat — seems to repeat itself in a most unpleasant beat!

The reason 60 to 70 million Americans continually diet, yet remain 62 percent overweight, is that diets have not conformed to people's lifestyles or food preferences. They aren't able to choose foods that make them feel happy. It's unreasonable to ask people to make radical changes in their behavior — to change their diet or style of living overnight.

We all need to stop labeling foods as good or bad. We need to begin to maximize our enjoyment, as well as our health. Otherwise we're likely to feel deprived or bored, resulting in overeating and abandoning programs. Since we know the trick usually isn't in losing weight, but rather keeping it off, the best way to reach and maintain a desirable body weight is to STOP DIETING!

Instead of dieting as such, it's better to eat smaller portions of all types of foods. Rather than cutting out all the foods you love, adopt a healthier perspective. Make positive changes in the way you think about food. Blend moderation, dietary discretion and good nutrition. All of this can be done with convenience foods. It's a matter of good nutrition. Cut back, not necessarily out!

Put Yourself in Charge!

Learning to modify your behavior and diet can lead to real changes in your weight. Take it from me. I was a heavy child, but I learned to follow a sensible eating program without giving up my favorite foods. Today, people call me skinny. They never believe me when I tell them I have, and always will have, a weight problem. The difference, however, is that the problem doesn't have me. I have control over it. You too can gain control! Wouldn't you rather have a little of something you liked than a plate full of food you didn't?

As you learn to eat smaller portions, it's very important to consider the "nutrient density" or nutritional composition of your total daily intake. In other words, while you shouldn't regularly eat sweet, empty-calorie foods, you can have a sweet treat once in a while. However, most of your food should have a high proportion of nutrients to calories. Once again, try to avoid fried, breaded or battered foods, cut down on salt and high-sodium foods and find lower calorie substitutes for fatty foodstuffs.

Prudent menu planning is the dieter's next best friend to exercise. It's smart to eat most of your calories as complex carbohydrates and starches. Potatoes, pasta, corn, rice, breads and other starches have been unfairly tagged as high-calorie culprits. It's what goes on top that tips the scales.

Fats, such as butter, sour cream and gravy, above all other foods, should be restricted. They contain two and one-quarter times the calories per gram as carbohydrates or proteins. Why not try following the Chinese tradition? Eat lots of vegetables, rice and grains, and smaller portions of meat, poultry and seafood.

Experiment and explore the multitude of fresh, frozen and processed fruits, grains and vegetables. Plan meals around them as opposed to around meats.

Unsweetened plain fruits, starchy vegetables and enriched whole-grain breads, crackers and cereals should be the center of your menu plans.

Remember not to limit yourself in food choices. For instance, there are other lean white meats besides chicken, turkey and fish. Trimmed veal or pork won't send your body into calorie shock. And if meats, poultry and fish aren't your favorites, you can get your protein by eating legumes (peas and beans), eggs, dairy products and protein-rich spreads. It's fats and simple sugars you need to curb. Foods such as bacon, olives, nuts, honey, jam and jellies should be kept to a minimum.

You Need the Basic Six

Healthy dining has long been viewed far too simplistically. Some define it as eating a combination of foods from the familiar Food Guide Pyramid recommendations. There is, however, much more to this system than meets the eye. The trick remains in learning how fats, sugars, combination dishes and desserts, which are not part of these guidelines fit into menu plans. Moreover, foods are groups including only partial listings of foods Americans typically consume.

Would you know how to account for fats such as margarine, oil or salad dressing, simple sugars from processed foods or combination dishes in your menus? Probably not, because they haven't been given a spot on the ever familiar "Guide to Good Nutrition." As a result, dieters don't always understand how a pat of butter, a grilled burger with cheese or even a drizzle of honey fits into a meal plan. It's also hard for people to break down combination items into food groups. How do you exchange or substitute foods when trying to eat light and right?

This is where *The Expresslane Diet* proves so advantageous! This program not only shows you how to incorporate Food Guide Pyramid recommendations, but it also provides the best examples of how to make convenience foods healthy. Even specialty calorie-reduced desserts are included. All selections provide variety, good taste and appeal without adding excess calories, cholesterol, fat, sodium or sugar. Moreover, to gain a more thorough understanding of food composition, *The Expresslane Diet* Exchange System and maintenance program introduce the dieter to six Basic Food Groups. You can learn to eat right without giving up the joy of eating.

The Expresslane Diet balances the U.S. RDAs for adults without exceeding needs for protein, fat, cholesterol, sodium and calories. Let's examine some of the individual components of dieting to better understand the "Basics" of healthy eating in the fast food lane.

Power Packed Proteins

Perhaps it's because we have long associated the mark of a man or woman by the cut of his or her meat that many Americans have grown accustomed to gorging on two to three times their daily quota of protein.

Proteins, however, are derived from a host of foods other than meat, fish or poultry. Starchy vegetables and grains including pasta, rice, bulgar, whole wheat or rye products contribute to our bodys' protein stores. In addition, milk and dairy products are protein-packed foods.

There are important differences to understand when selecting between animal and vegetable sources of protein. These two major classes of proteins are categorized as complete and incomplete proteins, respectively. Complete proteins are derived from most animal products such as pork, beef or poultry. They provide high biological value (HBV). HBV simply means these proteins contain all the essential amino acids our bodies do not manufacture. Vegetables and grains — unless appropriately combined — contain incomplete protein and do not provide HBV. If they are combined properly, however, vegetable and grain mixtures such as corn and soybeans can supply necessary complimentary essential amino acids to form HBV proteins. Roughly two-thirds of our daily protein consumption should be in the form of HBV proteins to provide the necessary stores of essential amino acids.

Since proteins can't be stored by the body, they should be consumed each day. However, more does not necessarily mean better. In the case of proteins, it's wise to guard against overconsumption, since excess protein can promote bone loss. It also taxes our kidneys and liver in making and breaking of by-products such as urea. Also, excesses may result in long-term health problems including obesity and atherosclerotic heart disease.

How much is enough protein for adults? Needs for dietary protein vary with age, sex and ideal body weight. An average adult between the ages of 22 and 59 years needs 44 to 56 grams per day for women and men, respectively. Between 12 and 20 percent of an adult's calories should be in the form of protein.

An easy rule of thumb when trying to translate grams of protein into portion sizes is to count each ounce serving of meat, poultry, fish or cheese as 7 grams of protein, 8 ounces of milk as 8 grams of protein, and breads, crackers, cereals or starchy vegetables at an average of 2 to 3 grams of protein per one-half cup serving. Foods that don't contain any appreciable protein include fats such as cream cheese, gravy or salad dressing and fruits or pure sugar.

Meeting Daily Needs

An adult woman could meet her daily protein needs of 44 grams by eating as little as 3 ounces of lean meat, drinking two 8-ounce glasses of low-fat milk or another equivalent dairy product, and 2 to 3 one-half cup servings of grains or starchy vegetables. It is certainly not the same as sinking your teeth into a juicy 8-ounce Porterhouse steak dinner complete with all the trimmings, averaging a whopping 60 grams of protein.

Opponents of convenience foods continue to criticize them for containing too much protein. While this can be true, not everyone guzzles down a double- or triple-decker burger, deluxe, supreme or super sandwich with a large order of French fries and a double-thick malted milk. Let's face it. Kids aren't the only people opting for regular size sandwiches and entrees. Besides, today's health-conscious American demands more lean meat, fresh fruit, whole-grain breads and vegetables. They are very aware of calories — often bringing some "fruit and vegetable basics" along when dining out. Healthy appetites have posed more than a challenge for companies and chains selling packaged foods. Demand has indeed sparked introduction of a vast number of wholesome foods. Health is all in the choosing, which can hopefully translate into the loss of unwanted pounds.

The Expresslane Diet contains a wide variety of favorite, convenient, portion-controlled protein sources. Planned portion sizes meet RDAs for adults and suggested caloric percentage compositions. Protein approximates 18 percent of the daily food intake.

Emphasis has been placed on incorporating light brand-name and chain specialty products markedly lower in total fat, cholesterol, sodium and calories. This plan features broiled, baked and roasted poultry, seafood, beef, lamb and pork. You will also find many combination dishes and lightly dressed salads instead of plain chops, steaks, burgers or broilers you may have been used to eating on other diets.

Going Cosmopolitan

The food from many different lands is featured in this plan. I recommend trying Mexican food. Become familiar with beans, such as kidney, garbanzo, pinto and navy, which are both rich in protein and a valuable source of dietary fiber. They are also lower in total fat and calories than many sandwich meats. Moreover, they are higher in vitamins and minerals such as potassium and phosphorus.

The Chinese cuisine is another style of dining I recommend integrating into your lifestyle. The Chinese have long shown us creative ways of balancing our love for meat in mixtures of nutrient-dense vegetables, fruits and grains. Even if you are dining at a fast-food Chinese restaurant, you usually have the option of ordering lean beef, pork or fish dishes prepared without salty monosodium glutamate (MSG) or cornstarch thickeners. It makes sense to have a small bowl of whole grain rice — high fiber, low calorie, low sodium and filling — as opposed to thickeners or fried noodles.

On the American front, you can order foods other than the classic burger on a bun. Packaged chef salads or mixtures of greens topped with chicken chunks or shrimp, single slices of pizza, the 300-calorie stuffed spud or submarines topped with low fat turkey breast, shaved beef or tuna salad are options in the American fast-food kingdom. Other choices include the "UNBURGER" — a regular-sized hot roast beef sandwich, broiled fish or chicken patties or chili con carni or soup. Even though these selections have been around for a while, they never seem to receive the same hype as burgers, fries and hot apple pie.

Some fast-food rules to remember with proteins include avoiding high-calorie, sodium or fatty toppings on sandwiches or salads such as bacon, mayo, cheese or regular salad dressing. Use of these four items alone adds 270 calories, hiking a regular sized plain burger from 255 to 525 calories. Instead, use toppings such as horseradish, mustard, ketchup or steak sauce, adding a measly 7, 11, 15 and 18 calories per tablespoon, respectively. If you can plan ahead, bring your own packages of low-sodium, low-calorie condiments. They cost a bit more, but you're worth it!

Try to avoid all meat products containing more than 30 percent fat. By sticking to original size entrees and scraping the coating off of breaded entrees, you'll be saving extra calories and fat. Try exercising portion control by automatically cutting a large sandwich or entree in half or eating items open-faced after removing excess meats, bread and toppings. If it bothers you to look at food you shouldn't eat, have it bagged to save for another meal. The "out of sight, out of mind" idea often works.

If you like pizza, feel free to enjoy it. It happens to be one of America's healthiest, nutritionally complete foods, provided you leave off the pepperoni, sausage, anchovies and extra cheese. Order a slice or two of cheese pizza topped with vegetables such as mushrooms, green peppers and onions. One-fourth of a 10-inch thin-crusted pizza has just 180 calories.

Remember, you do have choices. You can ask to have your meal prepared without added salt and have sauces served on the side. You may have to wait 10 to 15 minutes to have it your way, but that's all right. If companies perceive a demand for a given food or method of preparation, it's likely they'll give it a try. After all, demand spells dollars, which is the bottom line in any business.

In *The Expresslane Diet*, foods that are fried, dipped, sauced or blanketed are specially prepared without excess fats, cholesterol, sodium and calories. The undressed natural subtle flavors shine through as opposed to the stale deep-fat fried, cholesterol-rich, high-calorie mouthful you sometimes long for. Taste hasn't been sacrificed in the recipe modifications. In fact, flavor and taste rate high among consumers using products from this plan. For example, would you feel tastefully deprived dining on entrees of colorful pasta shapes stuffed with crab or shrimp, linguini laced in clam, scallop or marinara sauce, and spaghetti nuzzled between sweet bell peppers and Italian sausage? Other featured entrees include chicken chow mein, stir-fried or oriental beef with pea pods and rice and turkey divan. In addition, you can enjoy otherwise forbidden foods including subs, pizza and filled croissants. Gooey vegetables, sandwich toppings, chili, lasagna and stuffed pita pockets are also dished up in *The Expresslane Diet* program.

Fat's Where It's At

Fats count because th y are calorically two and one-quarter times more dense per gram than either carbohydrate or protein, and consequently must be restricted to lose weight. However, just as we have learned to substitute diet soft drinks for regular, so too can we begin to make appropriate fat substitutions.

Among the 10,000 new food products appearing annually on supermarket shelves, the number of reduced-fat and low-calorie items is remarkable. We can now substitute up to 98 percent of meats, including mock turkey products for regular ham, bologna and corned beef, and low-fat all-beef hot dogs. These products are low in cholesterol and fat. Some of the leaner options include lite cheeses, water-packed, low-fat tuna, salmon or chicken chunks, reduced calorie and fat marinades and salad dressings and frozen low-fat delights of ice milk, sorbet, yogurt and fresh fruit bars.

The word "fat" seems to cause negative feelings, as does the word "diet." How do you feel about it? Think it over. If you were overweight as a child, you were probably harassed. You might even have received elephant cards in your box on Valentine's day. Both socially and for your health, whether you are a child or an adult, fat is definitely not where it's at. Isn't it amazing that such a simple word carries so many overtones?

Though the word doesn't sound like it could taste good, fat is precisely what lends the most aroma, texture and taste to our foods. Unfortunately, along with enhancing food flavors, fats quickly add extra pounds and raise your risk of heart disease and cancer.

It's much easier to eat too many fats, as opposed to carbohydrates or protein. One pound of pure fat contains more than 4,000 calories, compared to just over 1,800 in an equal portion of carbohydrates or protein. So be careful about the quantity and quality of fats you eat. Exercising caution, however, doesn't mean reducing dietary fat to a level that jeopardizes good health.

Americans are getting the message about eating more fiber, starch, fish and poultry. Cutting back on total fats and cholesterol, if not properly monitored can leave you lacking in key nutrients. For instance, in an effort to decrease fat consumption, many Americans exclude red meat and eat fewer dairy products. This can lead to inadequate intake of folic acid, iron, zinc, vitamin B6, magnesium or calcium. Diets that are low in these nutrients may increase the risk of long-term nutritional problems, such as anemia and osteoporosis.

Despite bad press, fats are essential nutrients. They help to protect vital organs from injury, provide insulation against temperature extremes and supply energy for muscles. In addition, they help build regulatory substances, such as prostaglandins, that help regulate the body's use of cholesterol. More importantly, without dietary fats, transport and absorption of fat-soluble vitamins A, D, E and K would never occur.

About Fats

The three major types of fats are polyunsaturated, monounsaturated and saturated fatty acids. If you are trying to control cholesterol, today's buzz word is monounsaturates — olive oil, canola oil, peanuts, peanut oil. These three examples of this fatty acid purportedly increase the amount of good cholesterol — high density lipoprotein or HDL. Controlling cholesterol definitely involves lowering the amount of animal products you consume.

Some people mistakenly believe that a food labeled cholesterol-free is also low in saturated fat. The fact is many cholesterol-free products contain large amounts of saturated fatty acids — culprits that raise blood cholesterol. Many consumers are also confused about "hydrogenated" fats or oils. When a fat becomes hydrogenated, it merely becomes more saturated. And remember, it's the saturated fats that raise blood cholesterol. Therefore, even if you are using a polyunsaturated fat such as sunflower, safflower or corn oil, some of the cholesterol-lowering effects are cancelled by the hydrogenating process. It is a good idea to purchase whipped polyunsaturated margarine. It's better for your health and easier to spread on your toast. You can also use a little more.

Public health experts continually remind us of the link between saturated fats and cholesterol and an increased risk of heart disease. While some groups advocate an equal division of types of fats — a third in polyunsaturated, a third in monounsaturated and the remaining third in saturated fatty acids — the American Heart Association emphasizes the importance of the total amount of fat as a percentage of one's daily calories.

Typically, Americans consume approximately 40 percent of their daily calories as fats. Adults need only 10 percent for optimal functioning. That translates to a daily need as little as one tablespoon of fat. In other words, one tablespoon of margarine, mayonnaise or salad dressing daily is enough fat to supply your body with essential fatty acids.

Dietary recommendations from the American Heart Association and the American Cancer Society are somewhat more liberal. Fats are capped at a maximum 30 percent of daily calories. The importance of this recommendation is twofold: we should not only limit total fats to 30 percent of daily calories, but also, we need to restrict any type of foods containing more than 30 percent fat calories.

It's not difficult to determine your daily percentage of fat calories or the percentage of fat in a given food. Let me briefly acquaint you with the steps involved in both of these procedures. They're tools that should prove valuable in your quest to control your weight.

The percentage of daily fat calories is determined by an easy proportion. Steps are as follows:

Step 1: Multiply the number of fat calories by 100.

Step 2: Divide the result from Step 1 by the total number of daily calories.

Let's review an example. If you consume a daily total of 1,400 calories with approximately 600 calories of fat, what is the percentage of daily fat calories?

Step 1: 600 x 100 = 60,000

Step 2: 60,000 divided by 1,400 = 43% fat calories

Note: This percentage is 13 percentage points over the recommended cap of 30 percent fat calories.

The three easy steps to follow to determine the percentage of fat calories in any given foods are as follows:

Step 1: Multiply the number of grams of fat in a product by the number 9. This figure provides the total number of fat calories in a food. (The number 9 is used because there are 9 calories in each gram of fat)

Step 2: Take the result from Step 1 and multiply it by 100.

Step 3: Divide the result from Step 2 by the total number of calories. This figure gives you the percentage of fat calories per serving.

Let's review another example. If a piece of frosted chocolate devil's food cake contains a total of 233 calories with 11 grams of fat, what is the percentage of fat calories in this food?

Step 1: 11 x 9 = 99 fat calories

Step 2: 99 x 100 = 9,900

Step 3: 9,900 divided by 233 = 42% fat calories.

Note: This percentage is 12 points higher than we should typically consume.

After you have determined these values, there's yet another major point to consider. It's the difference between dietary fat and body fat. Dietary fat should only be equated with daily needs. Body fat, on the other hand, not only reflects dietary intake, but also includes consumption of excess proteins and carbohydrates. You can gain body fat even if you don't eat a single ounce of dietary fat. Too much protein, carbohydrate or fat leads to more stored body fat. That's why persons on low-calorie diets, taking in less energy or calories than their bodies need, lose body fat.

As you age, your proportion of body fat increases. At the same time, you also lose lean muscle mass. In fact, on average a 20-year-old woman's body is 26.5 percent fat. By age 35, her body fat has increased by nearly one-fourth to 33 percent body fat.

Fat tissue uses calories at a slower rate than muscle tissues. Since the ratio of fat to muscle increases as we age, we tend to burn fewer calories and store more fat. In other words, as we get older we can gain weight even if we consume the same number of calories. To counteract this biological fate, adults should restrict fatty food intake.

Controlling dietary fat involves restricting intake of familiar spreadable, shakable or pourable fats such as butter, oil, salad dressing or whipped cream cheese. Fatty cuts of beef or pork such as ribs or T-bone steak, processed cheese made with whole-milk bases and other high-fat dairy products, gravies, sauces, French fried foods, nuts, chocolate and baked goods in general are all sources of "hidden" fat. Some processed food contains as much as 85 percent fat calories per serving! That's why it's so important to read food labels and compare values, using other formulas for determining percentage fat calories.

Unfortunately, all fast foods continue to be given a bad rap when it comes to containing excess fat and cholesterol. Many health professionals claim fats and excess proteins are the major source of calories in fast-food meals. In fact, it all depends on what and how much you select! It's not the regular-sized burgers, sandwiches or salad bars that are bad; it's portions and everything extra that's added to them. It's the extra cheese, bacon, high-fat, high-calorie salad dressings and condiments, butter-based biscuits or croissants and sandwich fillings that add incredible amounts of fat and calories.

French fried entrees or side dishes drenched in gravy or butter also add insult to an otherwise lean piece of fish, chicken or potato. An Extra Crispy chicken breast contains 285 calories compared to 199 calories in the same piece of Original Recipe. The person opting for a French fried chicken dinner complete with roll, mashed potatoes, gravy and regular soda is eating 1,100 calories, nearly one-half of an adult man's daily calorie needs.

Many of the nation's 11,000 chicken and fish specialty fast-food restaurants do provide a lighter choice. Grilled or broiled chicken and fish are available at many fast-food spots. Low-fat fillers include fresh undressed salads, plain corn on the cob, mashed or baked potato without gravy and whole-grain rolls with margarine. And if per chance you're at a place where no other choice besides French fried exists, you can always remove the breading and fat and eat the meat.

Total fat and cholesterol in *The Expresslane Diet* approximates 22 grams of fat and less than 200 milligrams of cholesterol per day. That means on average, only 22 percent of this diet's daily calories come from fat. As a bonus, inclusion of high-fiber accompaniments, such as fresh fruits, vegetables and whole-grain products, makes this plan relatively high in dietary fiber. Fiber-rich foods also supply ample amounts of potassium — an important electrolyte.

Animal studies show that potassium from high-fiber fruits and vegetables may help protect arteries from the ravages of high blood pressure and lower the risk of stroke. Dietary fiber may also protect against cardiovascular disease by lowering blood cholesterol. Additionally, fiber foods provide some protection against colon and rectal cancer, help relieve constipation and slow the rate of glucose absorption by slowing gastric emptying time.

Fiber seems to "naturally" aid weight loss. By absorbing water and forming the necessary bulk within the digestive system, fiber leaves you feeling fuller. Since high-fiber foods are generally low in calories, one tends to feel fuller on fewer calories, which helps lose weight!   Total dietary fiber in *The Expresslane Diet* averages a generous 20 grams per day. To date, while no RDA exists for fiber, the National Cancer Institute and the American Cancer Society suggest that Americans double their current average daily intake of 12 grams to between 20 and 30 grams of fiber per day.

Suger Cues — The Bittersweet Facts Are Out

Though the concepts are hardly revolutionary, it's important to remember the following points:

1. Sugar is sugar, regardless of whether you are eating raw, refined, processed or natural.

2. Sugars are not nutrient dense. They provide nothing more than calories — 4 calories per gram.

3. Sugar is America's leading food additive; we typically consume 10 times more sugar than any other food additive with the exception of sodium. The average American consumes 24 percent of daily calories as sugar — amounting to as much as 128 pounds of sugar per person per year.

4. Sugars are added to foods for various reasons, including sweetness, moisture retention, prevention of spoilage and improved taste.

5. The most popular form of sugar is sucrose. Sweeteners account for approximately 18 percent of daily sugar calories. Manufacturers are permitted to add sucrose in unlimited quantities to some foods because, as a food additive, sucrose is on the "generally recognized as safe" (GRAS) list. The Senate Select Committee on Nutrition and Human Needs recommends that carbohydrates account for 55 to 60 percent of daily calories. They suggest that the portion of calories from simple refined white sugar or processed sugars be dropped from the current 18 percent to 10 percent. In other words, most carbohydrates should be from complex sources, such as potatoes, legumes and whole grains, or naturally occurring sugars in fruits and vegetables. It goes without saying that carbohydrates shouldn't be covered with fatty toppings.

6. Even if you never see the white crystals, they are crystal clear in thousands of processed foods. It's simply a matter of analyzing labels. Hidden sugars such as corn syrup, corn syrup solids, corn sugar, maple syrup, molasses and honey abound in packaged goods. Some cereals, packaged pudding, cake or stuffing mixes, seasonings, condiments, sauces, ice cream, regular soft drinks and candy are a few examples of sugar-laden foods.

7. The two basic types of sugars include monosaccharides such as glucose, fructose and galactose, and disaccharides in the form of sucrose, lactose and maltose. Read labels carefully and avoid purchasing a product if sugar in any form is among the top three ingredients listed on a food label.

8. Foods we tend to think of as wholesome, such as granola, aren't necessarily low in sugar. They often have corn syrup solids, saturated fats and honey added. Here's another case where labels tell the story.

9. To tally the exact amount of sugar in a given food, divide the number of grams of sugar by four. This number gives you the teaspoons of sugar in a product.

10. In order not to cry the sugar blues, you can eat less sugar by following these suggestions:

- Eat more complex carbohydrates such as fruit, vegetables and whole grains.

- Cut out empty-calorie junk food, such as regular candy, soft drinks, cakes and cookies.

- Restrict your consumption of fruit drinks or juices to only those prepared without added sugar. A 12-ounce regular fruit-flavored soft drink contains 4 tablespoons of sugar!

- Avoid regular consumption of alcohol — beer, wine and spirits.

- When you are looking to satisfy your sweet tooth without adding excess fat, cholesterol or sodium, fruit is always a great choice. You can use fresh, frozen or canned unsweetened as well as dried fruits. After dicing, slicing or cutting in half, you can bake, broil or stew fruits in addition to enjoying them in their raw natural state.

■   Try making your own desserts or purchasing low-fat, low-calorie, low-sugar treats.   When used in moderation, sugar substitutes, such as aspartame, are not harmful to your health.

The Expresslane Diet is naturally low in sugar.   Menus include a variety of low-sugar jams, jellies, spreads, brown and white sugar substitutes, diet waffle or pancake syrup and reduced-calorie desserts low in sugar.   This plan is complete with complex sugars including whole grains, cereals, breads, bagels, pancakes and starchy vegetables.

Sodium Secrets

In the 1970s, people were hard pressed to find low-sodium substitutes for favorites foods.   Now, the market has changed. Regardless of your preference for processed, convenience, ready-made, frozen or fast foods, you have lots of choices.

Foods formerly considered high in sodium such as pickles, condiments, canned soups, processed cheeses, fish and meat products, snacks and crackers are all available in low-sodium versions.   Requests for foods prepared without added salt are usually honored in both gourmet and fast-food restaurants.

For many people, the thought of a change in taste or lack of familiar food flavors is a difficult adjustment.   However, salt is a learned taste you can learn to do without.   Some people salt their food before they even taste it.   Remember the "trade offs."   If you prefer to eat convenience foods you know have been salted before cooking, you shouldn't add salt at the table.   Each teaspoon of table salt contains approximately 2,300 milligrams of sodium.

The Senate Select Committee on Health and Human Needs and other professional health groups recommend Americans consume 2,400 milligrams or less sodium per day. Since almost all foods contain sodium, with the exception of certain bottled waters and fruits, it stands to reason you would never have to use a salt shaker.   Most people's craving for salt seems to disappear in about a month.   This is a small price to pay for a lower risk of high blood pressure and stroke.

If you're concerned you won't be getting enough dietary sodium, fear not.   Deficiencies are exceedingly rare.   Considering only

500 milligrams of sodium are needed for optimum health, a small bowl of cereal with milk and a slice of toast with margarine provides almost all you need — 470 milligrams. If that seems hard to believe, check out the foods you love in a book such as Barbara Kraus's *Complete Guide to Sodium.*

Dietary sodium in *The Expresslane Diet* registers well below the suggested daily maximum of 2,400 milligrams per day. Daily averages approximate 2,000 milligrams for women and 2,300 milligrams for men.

Fast food meals can easily contain 75 percent of your daily sodium needs if foods are salted during preparation or if salty pickles, condiments, cheeses, bacon, olives or croutons are added.

Let's examine average sodium contents of a few favorite fast foods.

- Burgers range between 900 and 1,000 milligrams of sodium.
- Roast beef or fish sandwiches range from 700 to 900 milligrams.
- Chili with soda crackers has 1,100 to 1,300 milligrams.
- Grilled chicken breast sandwich has 600 to 700 milligrams.
- Chef salad has about 850 milligrams of sodium.
- A Chinese dinner averages 1,200 milligrams.
- A frosty milkshake or slice of pie averages 300 to 400 milligrams of sodium, respectively.

Some General Rules to Restrict Sodium in the Convenience or Fast Food Lane

1. Try to restrict any foods that provide more than one-third of your daily sodium needs. In other words, avoid any food with more than 800 milligrams of sodium.

2. When dining out, request foods prepared without salt. You may have to wait an extra 15 minutes for the next batch of burgers or fries, but it's a small price to pay for your health.

3. Hold the pickle, hold the relish, mustard, ketchup and all other condiments. In a fast-food spot, limit yourself to one small single packet of ketchup, horseradish or mustard per sandwich, unless you are using a special low-sodium variety.

4. Become familiar with the market's array of dry herbs, spices and condiments prepared without added salt. Think of it in a fun way — perhaps experimenting with different spice combinations each week.

5. When you place your order, request sauces on the side. Use any and all of them sparingly, since their bases are often salty broth, ketchup, tomato sauce or cheese. Many low-sodium sauces are available, including soy sauce, barbeque sauce and tomato sauce. Remember to also avoid sauces high in both fat and salt such as cheese or cream sauces.

6. Limit the amount of bacon bits, salad dressing, seasoned croutons, salted nuts, processed shredded cheeses or meats you use at the salad bar. Flavored vinegars, low-sodium vegetable juices mixed with herbs, freshly squeezed lemon or lime juice, ground pepper or red pepper flakes and low sodium salad dressings can all be used to boost flavors. Many products are low in calories, fat and sodium. Again and always, it's a matter of analyzing the food labels.

7. Low-calorie, low-sodium dressings can be purchased in single packets that easily fit into your purse, pocket or briefcase. Or you can carry small amounts of condiments or dressings in mini-containers. There's no more room for rationalizing.

8. Try adding a little wine when cooking—limited to 1/4 cup per day.

9. When a convenience product calls for adding broth or margarine, use the low-sodium varieties of broth and flavor with dried herbs.

10. If cooking directions call for adding salt during cooking, leave it out.

11. Limit consumption of baked goods. Baking soda and baking powder contain appreciable amounts of sodium.

12. When a low-sodium convenience entree exists, buy it and give it a try.

13. Examine canned goods and shelf-stable entrees! You can choose low-sodium canned vegetables, tuna, salmon, chicken chunks, both creamed or broth-based soups and sauces for all types of dishes. You don't have to pay premium prices; numerous generic and name-brand low-sodium options exist. A 6 1/2-ounce can of water-packed tuna or a cup of regular chicken noodle soup contains as much as 1,100 and 840 milligrams of sodium, respectively. Some of the latest shelf-stable entrees have more than 1,600 milligrams of sodium per serving. The figures add up quickly.

14. Limit both regular and calorie-reduced deli meats, cured meat products and cheese: It makes salt sense to restrict consumption of ham, bologna, salami, hot dogs, processed cheese or semi-soft spreads. A single ounce of regular deli meat averages 300 milligrams of sodium and cheese provides 315 milligrams of sodium per ounce. Some of the calorie-and fat-reduced deli products have more sodium than the regular versions, containing as much as 450 milligrams of sodium per ounce. Few of us make sandwiches with just 1 ounce of meat or cheese.

15. Carefully select packages of convenience foods. Check the label and be sure to plan amounts into your menus. Don't add extra salt or a seasoning blend containing salt to these "helpers."

Chapter 5

Tips for Staying On Top

If you eat sensibly, exercise in moderation and are a disciplined eater, you can stay slim forever. More importantly, if you can learn to modify your behavior, you will feel as great as you look.

Once you have reached your desired body weight, the hard work first begins. You must continue to eat sensibly by incorporating a balance of key nutrients, variety and moderation. In other words, dieting does not begin and end once you reach your goal weight. You can't return to previous food patterns or you will surely regain the weight you lost.

Although you may not be eating more food, weight gain may occur over the years because of the body's natural tendencies. After age 25, adults gain an average of one pound of body fat per year. While this might not sound like a lot of weight, by age 40 a svelte, 125-pound woman could tip the scales at 140 without having changed her eating patterns. In order to turn this around, you need to continually examine calories and overall food composition.

In this chapter we'll review tips on how to maintain weight, modify food-related behaviors without the pain associated with fitness or exercise regimens.

Behavior Modification

One of the most difficult things to change is your behavior, particularly if it involves food. After all, you've been eating all of your life. The eating patterns you have today are a direct result of what you've learned since infancy.

Eating patterns are often unconscious. You are unaware of what you eat, when you eat, how much you eat and why you eat it. Moreover, sometimes your appetite — real or imagined —

rather than hunger stimulates consumption. External food cues, such as the sight of a buffet, the smell of fresh baked goodies or a glimpse of a picture of your favorite dessert, can also stimulate appetite and trigger a desire to eat. Additionally, internal cues such as your mood can promote a desire to eat. Have you ever noticed that you overeat when you are stressed, lonely or anxious? This is sometimes called the "mood-feeding connection."

The trick to effective self-control is becoming aware of eating patterns — the "chain" of events that set your appetite on automatic pilot. By modifying the links in your chain of behaviors and replacing them with positive new behaviors, you can "unlearn" old habits and establish new ones. Behaviors are patterned as follows:

T_____ B_____ R_____
TRIGGER -------- BEHAVIOR ------- RESULT

Example:

HUNGER --------- EAT ------------- SATISFACTION
                                   (SATIETY)

Since the result of this example is a positive one — relief of hunger and satisfaction — it acts to positively reinforce the preceeding behavior. Because your eating behaviors have been getting positive reinforcement for many years, your goal will be to "unlearn" old habits that trigger appetite and observe the T-B-R chain of events to establish new eating behaviors.

Behavior modification is a simple, measurable technique that, when mastered, can provide you with the necessary tools to change your eating habits. It has been used for years to promote successful weight reduction and maintenance. As it is a personalized method, you and you alone decide what habits you need to change and how to reshape them to fit your lifestyle.

The first step in gaining control is to become aware of current habits. You not only need to know the triggers or why you eat, but also, how often, how fast and how much you eat.

One of the best ways to evaluate food habits is by keeping a daily food diary. By honestly and faithfully writing down what you put into your mouth and what your activity is, you will discover after a month or two, which habits are automatic and which are by choice. For example, do you sit down to eat lunch because it's noon and you are bored? Do you always eat when you're preparing dinner, watching television or talking on the telephone? Are you a closet eater? Do you reward yourself with food if you had a great day or feel you earned it?

By becoming aware of the activities and moods that set off your emotional appetite, you can break reflex habits and find different activities to take the place of eating. For instance, try doing something that is incompatible with eating like chewing sugarless gum, jumping rope, singing a song or taking a hot shower. Practice or rehearse new behaviors. Imagine how you would like to eat, and then go through the actions as if you were rehearsing for a theatrical performance. Practice saying, "No thank you. I'm not hungry." Use smaller plates so that food portions appear larger. If coming through the kitchen door and seeing the refrigerator sets your appetite off, enter the house from the front door. Eat only while sitting in one place at the kitchen or dining room table. Put down your silverware between bites and talk with your dining companion. It's amazing how satisfying and filling, yet calorie-free conversation can be.

A sample diary is shown on the next two pages. After you've completed your diary for one week, try to identify one or two problem eating behaviors. After a month, try to identify patterns of problem eating behaviors. Then, list the possible triggers or cues, jotting down possible suggestions for modifying your behavior on the "chain."

You may find that TV commercials for pizza send you to the telephone for a pizza delivery or a Coca Cola fix. Are you surprised when you are unable to stop at the taste of one sweet treat and you wind up devouring the entire package of cookies or candy? In these situations, the triggers are as simple as television commercials and keeping "high-risk" favorite foods in the house. The "out of sight, out of mind" theory often conquers the problem.

To effectively deal with triggers, all you have to do is set a plan of attack. One method that has proven helpful is the A-C-E method, where you Arrange, Control and Eliminate the trigger. For instance, you arrange to watch television without commercial breaks and eliminate purchasing favorite empty-calorie sweet treats. To control the trigger, you repeat your resolve to avoid eating sweets as you pass the bakery aisle in the supermarket. By simply letting your creativity guide you, you can A-C-E the problem!

SAMPLE FOOD DIARY

MEAL/SNACK Time of Day Time Spent Eating	ACTIVITY/ PLACE	FOOD/BEV. CONSUMED	AMOUNTS (APPROX.)	MOOD (CUES)	EXERCISE/ Min. Spent
BREAKFAST					
____ a.m./p.m.	_____	_____	_____	_____	_____
____ min/hr	_____	_____	_____		_____
		_____	_____		
		_____	_____		
		_____	_____		
SNACK					
____ a.m./p.m.	_____	_____	_____	_____	_____
____ min/hr	_____	_____	_____		_____
LUNCH					
____ a.m./p.m.	_____	_____	_____	_____	_____
____ min/hr	_____	_____	_____		_____
		_____	_____		
		_____	_____		
		_____	_____		
SNACK					
____ a.m./p.m.	_____	_____	_____	_____	_____
____ min/hr	_____	_____	_____		_____
DINNER					
____ a.m./p.m.	_____	_____	_____	_____	_____
____ min/hr	_____	_____	_____		_____
		_____	_____		
		_____	_____		
		_____	_____		
SNACK					
____ a.m./p.m.	_____	_____	_____	_____	_____
____ min/hr	_____	_____	_____		

SAMPLE FOOD DIARY

MEAL/SNACK Time of Day Time Spent Eating	ACTIVITY/ PLACE	FOOD/BEV. CONSUMED	AMOUNTS (APPROX.)	MOOD (CUES)	EXERCISE/ Min. Spent
BREAKFAST 7 (a.m.)/p.m. 10 (min)/hr	Watching TV Home Kitchen	Cheerios/ Cereal 2% Milk Banana Decaf c̄ Sugar	1½ C. 1 ½ C. 1 small 2 C./ 2 tsp.	Pressured	– –
SNACK 10 (a.m.)/p.m. 10 (min)/hr	Talking Office Cafeteria	Bran Muffin Decaf c̄ Sugar	1 med. 1 C./ 1 tsp.	Happy "In the swing of things!"	– –
LUNCH 12:30 a.m./(p.m.) 20 (min)/hr	Reading Newspaper Desk @ Work	"Sub Sandwich" {Fr. Bread {Tuna salad Lettuce Tomato Fresh Pear Mineral Water Fresh Lime	½ (4") roll ½ C. 2 leaves 2 slices 1 small 1 (12 oz) bottle 2 slices	Hungry	Walked/ 20 min.
SNACK 5:30 a.m./(p.m.) 15 (min)/hr	Driving Car In Auto	Oatmeal Cookie Coke	1 med 1 (12 oz) can	Restless	– –
DINNER 7:30 a.m./(p.m.) 2 min/(hr)	Talking Restaurant	White wine Tossed Greens Fr. Dressing Br. Chicken Gr. Beans Baked Potato Butter Fresh Raspberries Decaf c̄ Sugar	4 fl oz 1½ C. 2 Tbsp. 1 (3½ oz.) Breast ½ C. 1 med 2 Pats 3/4 C. 2 C. / 2 tsp	Relaxed	–
SNACK 11 a.m./(p.m.) 3 (min)/hr		2% Milk	½ C.	Tired	– –

Changing your reward system is as beneficial as changing your behavior to modify your present eating patterns. When you determine a reward, make it something other than food. It should also be something that is special to you. For instance, buy yourself a ticket to a sports spectacular, have your hair done, go for a body massage or take a luxurious bubble bath in a candlelit sunken tub.

When habits are new and positive, it is important that you reward yourself frequently — after each time you practice them. As the behavior becomes more routine, rewards can be given on an intermittent schedule. Chart your new behaviors to monitor your progress. For example, if your goal was to stop reading the newspaper while eating or taking at least 20 minutes to complete a meal, you can chart the number of days in a given week that you complied with it and reward yourself on a percentage basis. Set reasonable goals such as 75 percent compliance as opposed to 100 percent perfection. This will allow you to be challenged by your new behavioral goals without setting yourself up to fail against impossible odds.

Some other helpful behavioral changes include:

- Shop only from prepared lists.
- Shop only after eating.
- Set a pleasant place for yourself at the table (cloth, mats, napkins, flowers, candles, etc.).
- Deliberately set your fork down between bites.
- Don't eat off another person's plate.
- Don't sample food as you cook it.
- Don't finish leftovers as you're putting them away.
- Spoil any food that tempts you too strongly. (Throw it in the garbage can or disposal.)
- When eating, make that your only activity.
- Take at least 20 minutes to finish a meal.
- Keep all "high risk" foods out of the house or, if you have to treat yourself, buy a single serving.
- Stock the fridge and pantry with "free foods" so you have them as needed.
- Drink a glass of water before and after meals.

- Exercise before eating.
- Practice how to relax (music, quiet time alone, exercising, etc.).
- Gather support from a family member or friend.
- Keep a before and after picture of yourself on the fridge with notes about behaviors leading to overweight and positive changes.
- Plan your menu selections ahead whether you're dining at home or on the run.
- Call a restaurant ahead to confirm they have what you want and will prepare it the way you want it.
- Tell your host or hostess "No thank you" without feeling guilty.
- Keep daily food records even after you reach your goal weight — continuing to key into food triggers or cues.

While I don't encourage counting every single calorie that passes your lips, you should know approximately how many calories your body needs to maintain a desirable body weight range. One of the simplest ways to determine calorie maintenance needs is by the following three-step formula:

STEP 1: Multiply your height in inches by 3.5.

STEP 2: Subtract 108 from Step 1.

STEP 3: Multiply Step 2 by one of the following activity factors to determine the number of calories you need to maintain your weight:

X 14 for sedentary adults
X 15 for moderately active adults
X 16 for very active adults

Using this formula, let's take a look at an example: How many calories should a 5-foot, 4-inch woman, who is moderately active, consume to maintain her weight?

STEP 1: 64 inches X 3.5 = 224

STEP 2: 224 – 108 = 116

STEP 3: 116 X 5 = 1,740 calories

Answer: Approximately 1,740 calories

To avoid calorie counting or detailed calculations for grams of fat, carbohydrates and protein, separate food group Maintenance Minimum/Maximum Systems have been developed for men and women. Tables are based on selecting foods from the Basic Six Food Groups or continuing with *The Expresslane Diet* Exchange System.

Since each person requires a different amount of calories to maintain his or her weight and burns calories at a different rate, you will have to decide your body's unique MAXIMUM levels for any food group specifying a Minimum rather than a Maximum level.

Selected foods for Minimum/Maximum *Expresslane Diet* Exchanges match all rules discussed in the diet section of the plan. Rules for maintaining an "edge" with the Basic Six Guidelines follow.

Basic Six Guidelines:
Minimum and Maximum Food Allowances for Weight Maintenance

Maximums refer to cooked weight of meats such as lean poultry, beef, veal and pork. A single serving equals 1 ounce of cooked protein and approximates 55 to 73 calories. Weigh meats after cooking with all visible fat and skin removed. Permissible types and methods of preparation are the same as those listed in the rules for dieting.

All dairy products consumed must contain skim milk or low-fat bases. A single serving approximates 80 to 100 calories. Examples of single-serving equivalents include 1 ounce of low-fat cheese, 8 ounces of skim or buttermilk, 4 ounces of skimmed evaporated milk, 8 ounces of plain low-fat yogurt, 1/2 cup of low-fat cottage cheese, and 1/2 cup of low-fat frozen dessert, such as ice milk or yogurt.

Grains include plain, unfrosted breads, cereals, starchy vegetables, pasta and noodles. A single serving approximates 70 to 100 calories. Examples of single-serving equivalents include 1/2 cup of a cooked cereal or starch, such as pasta or rice, 1/2 cup of a starchy vegetable such as peas, potatoes, beans or corn, and 1-ounce servings of a bread product such as 1/2 a bun, 1 small muffin or 1 slice of toast. It's best to select whole-grain products enriched with iron.

Select fruits and vegetables containing vitamin C and A every day and every other day, respectively. Examples of vitamin C-containing fruits and vegetables include grapefruits, melons, tomatoes and carrots. Vitamin A sources include deep green or dark yellow vegetables such as broccoli, squash and beans. Single servings of fruits approximate 40 to 60 calories, compared with 25 to 40 calories in a serving of vegetables. The serving size for one serving of fruit is a small piece of fresh fruit or 1/4 cup dried or 1/2 cup of unsweetened, canned, processed or frozen fruit. Single servings of vegetables approximate 1/2 cup cooked or one cup raw. They should be prepared without added fat.

Each serving of fat approximates 45 to 60 calories. Be sure to measure fats carefully. Examples of single-serving equivalents include 1 teaspoon of margarine or mayonnaise, 1 tablespoon of regular or 2 tablespoons of diet salad dressing and 1 tablespoon of cream cheese. You can always use lower-fat varieties to get a little extra.

You will also find Basic Six Maintenance Bonus/Free Food Mates and Mixers, and a guide to incorporating "Formerly Forbidden Foods," such as alcohol and sweets. Remember to account for any foods added to the maintenance guidelines. Tally servings each day and be certain they don't exceed your calculated calories value.

Continue to avoid foods high in sodium and simple sugars, as well as fat, cholesterol and calories. In other words, the same principles practiced in *The Expresslane Diet* still apply. The major difference, however, is that you have more calories.

The following page provides daily Minimum/Maximum food guidelines for maintaining weight. The choice is yours — you can either opt to follow the Basic Six Daily Food Guide or *The Expresslane Diet* Exchange System for lasting weight control.

Basic Six Daily Maintenance Minimums and Maximums for Weight Control

Women 22 to 59 years of age

FOOD GROUP	MINIMUM	MAXIMUM
Meat		5 oz.
Milk/dairy	2 servings	
Grains	6 servings	
Fruits	3 servings	
Vegetables	3 servings	
Fats		4 servings
Free foods		Unlimited

Men 22 to 59 years of age

FOOD GROUP	MINIMUM	MAXIMUM
Meat		7 oz.
Milk/dairy	2 servings	
Grains	10 servings	
Fruits	5 servings	
Vegetables	3 servings	
Fats		4 servings
Free foods		Unlimited

System Maintenance Minimums and Maximums for Weight Control

Women 22 to 59 years of age

EXCHANGE GROUP	MINIMUM	MAXIMUM
For Beginners	1 serving	1 serving
Frozen Classics/ Convenience Entrees	1 serving	1 serving
Protein Pleasers	2 servings	3 servings
Fruits, Berries, Cherries & Much More	3 servings	4 servings
Vegetables Galore	3 servings	4 servings
Super Side Dishes	2 servings	2 servings
Milk Magic	2 servings	2 servings
Sauces Aside	1 serving	2 servings
Free Foods		Unlimited

Men 22 to 59 years of age

EXCHANGE GROUP	MINIMUM	MAXIMUM
For Beginners	1 serving	2 servings
Frozen Classics/ Convenience Entrees	1 serving	2 servings
Protein Pleasers	3 servings	3 servings
Fruits, Berries, Cherries & Much More	4 servings	5 servings
Vegetables Galore	4 servings	4 servings
Super Side Dishes	2 servings	3 servings
Milk Magic	2 servings	2 servings
Sauces Aside	2 servings	3 servings
Free Foods		Unlimited

Basic Six Bonus/Free Maintenance Food Mates and Mixers

A bonus food or beverage contains less than 20 calories per serving. While on maintenance, you are permitted two choices of any items in the following groups specifying a serving size. All other items may be consumed throughout the day as desired.

BEVERAGES/DRINKS:

Coffee — regular or decaf, hot or iced without added sugar (all flavors)

Tea — regular or decaf, hot or iced without added sugar (all flavors)

Club soda or carbonated water without added sugar (low-sodium preferred)

Mineral water or regular tap water

Sugar-free tonic (low-sodium preferred)

Sugar-free soda (all flavors) with no more than 4 calories or 1 gram of carbohydrate per 6-ounce serving

Sugar-free fruit flavored drinks (all flavors) with no more than 4 calories or 1 gram carbohydrate per 6-ounce serving

Fresh lemon or lime, 1 whole squeezed in water or soda per day

MEAL ACCOMPANIMENTS:

1/2 cup cooked unsweetened cranberry sauce

1 tablespoon sugar-free jam or jelly

1/2 cup plain unsweetened gelatin

1/2 cup cooked unsweetened rhubarb sauce
1 tablespoon sugar-free syrup
1/4 cup dry wine (to be used in cooking only)

SALAD FIXINGS:

(1 cup raw, separated or mixed)
Alfalfa sprouts
Cabbage
Celery
Chicory
Chinese cabbage
Cucumbers
Endive
Escarole
Fennel
Lettuce, all varieties
Mushrooms, raw
Parsley
Peppers, red, green or hot
Pickles, unsweetened, low-sodium dill (1 medium)
Radishes
Scallions
Spinach, raw
Watercress
Zucchini

SEASONINGS — SPICES AND HERBS:

Basil, fresh or dried
Bay leaf
Celery seed
Chili powder
Chives
Cinnamon
Cloves
Cumin seed
Curry
Dill
Garlic, fresh or powder
Ginger
Ginger root, fresh
Lemon pepper
Mint

Nutmeg
Onion powder
Oregano
Paprika
Parsley
Rosemary
Sage
Dehydrated vegetable flakes

FLAVORINGS AND EXTRACTS:

Almond
Butter
Lemon
Lime
Orange
Peppermint
Vanilla
Walnut

CONVENIENCE SEASONING MIXES:

Chili seasoning mix (1 teaspoon)
Hickory smoke salt (1 teaspoon)
Meatball or spaghetti seasoning mix (1 teaspoon)
Pizza seasoning mix (1 teaspoon)
Seafood seasoning mix (1 teaspoon)
Taco seasoning mix (1 teaspoon)

CONDIMENTS:

Catsup, low-sodium
Chili sauce (1 tablespoon)
Horseradish
Hot pepper sauce
Mustard, low-sodium
Soy sauce, low-sodium (1 teaspoon)
Sweet & sour sauce (1 tablespoon)
Tabasco sauce
Taco sauce (1 tablespoon)
Tomato paste, low-sodium
Tomato puree, low-sodium
Tomato sauce, low-sodium
Vinegar (all varieties)
Worcestershire sauce

MISCELLANEOUS "MADNESS":

Sugar-free hard candy (2 pieces)
Sugar-free chewing gum (5 sticks)
1 teaspoon baking powder or baking soda
2 tablespoons sugar-free non-dairy whipped cream topping
1/2 cup low-calorie cranberry juice
Nonstick spray coating
Sugar substitute (saccharine or aspartame)

The Formerly Forbidden Foods

Are you willing to give up fruits, vegetables, meats and starches for a seemingly small, delicious sweet treat? Once in a while, even the most disciplined eater deserves a "break." Here's a compilation of delectables with exchange equivalents.

Any of the following items may be enjoyed once every week.

"Formerly Forbidden Foods"
How Much Are They Worth to You?

ALCOHOLIC BEVERAGES:	EXCHANGE MATE EQUIVALENTS:
Beer, regular (12 fluid ounces)	1 grain + 2 fat
Beer, light (12 fluid ounces)	1 grain
Brandy, apricot (1 cordial glass)	1/2 grain + 1/2 fat
Distilled Liquor (1 fluid ounce)	2 fat

WINE:	
Champagne, 4-ounce wine glass	1/2 fruit + 1 fat
Port, 3 1/2-ounce wine glass	1 grain + 1 1/2 fat
Sauterne, 3 1/2-ounce wine glass	1/2 fruit + 1 fat
Vermouth, dry 3 1/2 ounces	3 fat
Vermouth, sweet 3 1/2 ounces	1 grain + 2 fat

SUGAR-SWEETENED BEVERAGES:	
Eggnog, nonalcoholic (8 fluid ounces)	1 low-fat milk + 1 grain + 3 fat + 1/2 fruit

Gatorade (12 fluid ounces)	1 fruit
Lemonade (8 fluid ounces)	1 1/2 fruit
Malted Milk (8 fluid ounces)	1 low-fat milk + 1 fruit + 2 fat
Punch, fruit flavored (8 fluid ounces)	2 fruits

DESSERTS:

Brownie, chocolate w/nuts & icing (1 sm.)	1 grain + 1/2 fat
Cream Puff w/ custard filling — 1	1/2 low-fat milk + 1 grain + 3 fat
Eclair w/ chocolate filling and whipped cream	1 grain + 5 fat
Quick Bread, any fruit or nut flavor (1/12th prepared bread)	2 grain + 1/2 fat

COOKIES:

Plain unfrosted (2 pieces)	1 grain + 1 fat
Gingersnaps (3 pieces)	1 grain

CAKES:

Angel Food Cake (1/12th cake)	2 grain
Cheesecake (1/8th cake)	2 fat + 1/2 meat + 1 1/2 fruits
Frosted Layer Cake (1/8th cake)	1 grain + 1 fruit + 2 fat
Frosted Cupcake (vanilla or chocolate) — 1	1 grain + 1 fat + 1 fruit
Custard, vanilla (1/2 cup)	1/2 low-fat milk + 1 grain + 1 fat

DOUGHNUTS:

Plain cake or yeast type — 1	1 grain + 1 fat
Chocolate covered — 1	1 grain + 1 1/2 fat
Jelly filled — 1	1 1/2 grain + 1 1/2 fat
Powdered Sugar — 1	1 grain + 1 fat

FROZEN TREATS:

Ice Cream, any flavor (1/2 cup)	1 grain + 2 fat
Ice Cream Drumstick — 1	1 grain + 2 fat + 1/2 fruit
Ice Cream Sandwich — 1	1 grain + 2 fat + 1 fruit
Ice Milk, any flavor (1/2 cup)	1 grain + 1 fat
Ice Cream Cone (sugar type) — 1	1/2 grain
Sherbet, any flavor (1/2 cup)	2 grain

Pudding Pop, frozen, any flavor — 1   1 grain
Popsicle, any fruit flavor — 1   1 1/2 fruit
Frozen Fruit Juice Bar, any flavor — 1 1 fruit

TOPPINGS FOR FROZEN TREATS:
Butterscotch (2 Tbsp)   1/2 grain + 1 fruit
Chocolate Fudge Topping (2 Tbsp)   1 grain + 1/2 fat
Strawberry Topping (2 Tbsp)   1 grain + 1/2 fruit
Pudding, chocolate or vanilla
   made with low-fat milk (1/2 cup)   1/2 low-fat milk + 1
                                          grain + 1 fat

PIES:
Custard filled (1/8th pie)   1 meat + 1 grain + 1
                                          fat + 2 fruit

Pecan Pie (1/8th pie)   2 grain + 2 1/2 fruit +
                                          1/2 meat + 4 fat

FRUITED PIES: (All 1/8th pie)
Apple   1 grain + 2 fruit + 2 fat
Banana Cream   1 grain + 1 fruit + 2 fat
Cherry   2 grain + 2 fruit + 2 fat
Chocolate Cream with Cherries   1 grain + 1 1/2 fruit +
                                          2 fat

ASSORTED CANDIES:
Butter Mints (14 pieces)   1 1/2 fruit
Fudge, chocolate with nuts (1 ounce)   1 1/4 grain + 1 fat
Granola Bar, unfrosted (1 bar)   1 grain + 1 fat
Hard Candy (6 discs)   1 fruit
Jelly Beans (10 pieces)   1 fruit
Marshmallows (3 large)   1 fruit
Milk Chocolate Candy Bar, plain
   (1 ounce)   1 grain + 2 fat
Raisins, chocolate covered (1 ounce)   1/2 grain + 1 fruit +
                                          1/2 fat

SNACKS:
Potato or Corn Chips (1 ounce)   1 grain + 2 fat
Tortilla Chips (1 ounce)   1 grain + 2 fat
Carmel Coated Popcorn (1 cup)   1 grain + 1 fruit + 2 fat
Cheesecurls (1 ounce)   1 grain + 2 fat

SPREADABLE EDIBLES:

Barbecue Sauce (1/4 cup)	1/2 grain
Brie Cheese (1 ounce)	1 meat + 1/2 fat
Caviar, Sturgeon — granular or pressed (1 rounded tsp)	1/2 meat
Cheese Sauce (2 Tbsp)	1/4 low-fat milk + 1 fat
Cheese Spread, processed — any flavor (1 Tbsp)	1/2 meat
Cream Sauce (2 Tbsp)	1/4 low-fat milk + 1 fat
Honey (1 Tbsp)	1/2 fruit
Salsa (1/4 cup)	1/2 fruit
Sweet and Sour Sauce (2 Tbsp)	1 fruit

The following additional tips should help you to maintain favorable control of your weight:

1. Integrate the same meal planning techniques you followed in the diet phase of *The Expresslane Diet* to maintain your loss. Plan daily menus around three nutritionally complete meals. Menus should include a wide variety of all types of foods, not exceeding maximum amounts of any food group. It is important not to skip any meals. However, if it's easier for you to snack instead of eating three squares, simply S T R E T C H recommended daily allowances over four to six small feedings each day.

2. Whether you're preparing a meal at home or eating out, plan menus around a balance of lean baked, broiled, roasted or poached meats. Go lightly on the added fats, simple sugars and sweets. Steer clear of casseroles, fried, battered or breaded foods and sauced concoctions.

3. Some easy rules of thumb to practice when eating out include:

   ■ Order exactly what you want — no more, no less.

   ■ Plan what you're going to order before you enter the restaurant. Make allowances for what you'll be ordering during the day. For instance, if you know you will be having a rather large dinner, eat a lighter breakfast and lunch. Save the calories.

   ■ If you don't see something on the menu you want, ask for it. Often the chef may prepare it at a slightly higher cost than regular menu items. Examples include special fresh fruits such as melons in season, a special cut of beef or type of fish dry broiled.

- Always request plain entrees, salads or meal compliments. Ask for sauces or condiments on the side.

- Keep a ready supply of low-calorie salad dressing, fresh fruit and crackers in small ready-to-serve packages. Think of this in a spirit of picnicking — packing a snack or meal accompaniment that's legal.

4. Weigh yourself once a week at the same time of day and in approximately the same type of clothing. If the scale registers a 3 to 5 pound gain in weight and if you have exceeded daily food group maximums on maintenance, cut back. If this isn't the case, resume *The Expresslane Diet* for at least one week or until you've returned to your desired weight.

5. Always remain informed. Keep a supplementary food guide listing nutritional information on all types of products as well as *The Expresslane Diet* Exchange System handy for comparing and substituting foods desired. Any food addition or deletion you make will influence nutritional balance, composition and calories. Also remember to refer back to the chapter on dietary principles or equivalents of grams of protein, carbohydrate and fats to determine appropriate food substitutions. For example, if you want to eat an entree containing 22 grams of protein and 10 grams of fat, you would understand that it supplies approximately three servings of meat and two of fat. Each ounce of meat equals 7 grams of protein, and 1 teaspoon of fat approximates 5 grams.

6. Request nutritional information wherever you dine, especially at fast-food restaurants. Ask how the food is prepared or about other concerns you may have. Request that food or preparation be changed when necessary.

7. Always read and reread food labels at the supermarket and select the market's best nutritional buy.

8. Bad habits are hard to break, but make an effort *not* to:

- Eat unconsciously.

- Eat when you are not hungry.

- Eat when you feel bored, angry, sad or depressed, happy, over anxious, etc.

- Eat leftovers from kid's or spouse's plates. Don't be a member of the Clean Plate Club. When you've had enough, wrap or take the rest home for another meal.

- Eat by the clock — it's noon so it's time for lunch — WRONG!

- Give into food cues such as smell, sight and taste.

- Eat a meal in less than 15 minutes.

- Live to eat instead of eat to live.

- Eat in places other than your designated dining area such as bed, while cooking, talking on the telephone or watching television.

- Rush through preparations for a meal. Make meals as simple or fancy as you want. Arrange flowers, candles, festive cloth and garnish foods.

9. Continue to avoid using a salt shaker at the table or when preparing foods. Whenever possible, purchase foods, condiments or beverages in low-sodium versions. Use permissible dry herbs, spices, unsweetened fresh fruit juices and a little wine in cooking to pick up food flavors. When dining out, request that foods be prepared without added salt.

10. Continue to purchase and use low-fat low-sugar substitutes, spreads, salad dressings and dairy products.

11. Continue to purchase foods without added sugars such as fruit juices, breakfast cereals, prepared mixes and jellies. Use sugar substitutes in moderation and try low-sugar modified products.

12. When you start your maintenance program, you should be able to guesstimate portions. If, however, you are uncomfortable doing this, weigh and measure foods. Be sure to use appropriate liquid and dry measures.

13. If in doubt about a given food, leave it out.

14. Don't consume alcohol, sweets or fatty foods regularly. On occasion, if you want a sweet treat or some alcohol, refer to the list of equivalent food values and calories for Formerly Forbidden Foods.

15. When cooking or ordering meals out, substitute low-sodium, low-fat and lower calorie foods whenever you can. Try modifying some of your favorite recipes to create healthier dishes.

16. Continue to drink at least four to six 8-ounce glasses of pure water each day. It's best to drink them right before sitting down to a meal. It helps you feel fuller.

Exercise to the Beat of a Renewed You

Does the thought of exercising with Cher or Jane Fonda leave you defeated before you begin? Let's face it, Mother Nature didn't make us all in the image of Arnold Schwarzenegger or Raquel Welch. Even exercising three to four times a week isn't going to give you a body like Bruce Jenner or Marilyn Monroe. On the contrary, if that were the case, liposuction, tummy, bust or buttocks tucking, hormonal injections and the like would never have stood the test of time. Exercise experts, promising chests like Victoria Principal's and waists like Vivian Leigh's without proper diet are more like "Gone With the Wind."

Sometimes just the thought of exercising might tire you out. But that need not be the case if you understand exercise doesn't necessarily involve strenuous work. Bar bells, tummy crunchers and weight lifting equipment aren't the only means to becoming fit as a fiddle. You need not be a marathon racer either. The whole fitness arena has become far too sophisticated for many. It's time to shift gears from the dream world of gorgeous bodies to the acceptance of reality.

In spite of the number of health and fitness clubs available to us, Americans are not in better shape than before the fitness craze began. Those bicyclists, runners and walkers you see parading shopping malls, trails and tracks are the exception to the rule. According to a 1986 survey by the U.S. Department of Health and Human Services, more than 80 percent of Americans don't even get the minimum amount of exercise recommended by the American Heart Association, which is half an hour of aerobic (oxygen-using) exercise at least three times a week. The professionals are telling us we should exercise each day. In fact, some studies show that daily exercise produces extra benefits compared with exercising three times a week. While anything in extreme can be detrimental, Americans who exclude rather than restrict types of activities, risk body burn-out and poor health.

Lack of exercise usually is linked with lack of time, busy lifestyles and long work days. Some Americans don't view exercise as remedial medicine or preventive health care. Exercise is not quite up there with quitting cigarette smoking, decreasing saturated fat and cholesterol or eating more fiber and starch. A final reason why Americans don't get out and play stems from physical limitations, including bad knees, joints or respiratory problems.

Resting metabolism, often referred to as basal metabolic rate (BMR), declines by 10 percent per decade after the age of 25. Without exercise, an average 35-year-old man can gain up to one-third of a pound of fat per year until age 60. That's a difference of 8 1/4 pounds of fat. As we age, it's important to find ways to burn extra calories to maintain our weight. The answer is not a matter of limiting oneself to dieting.

Exercise is beneficial not only because it burns calories and speeds BMR, but also because it helps reduce appetite, burn fat, trim inches and build lean muscle mass. Also, exercise fosters a positive self-image and helps to kick chronic fatigue that has no physical basis. More importantly, studies suggest that aerobic activities in particular may reverse heart damage caused by high blood pressure, thereby cutting the risk of heart attack.

Today's exercisers have wide choices for calorie burn offs. They can opt for impact or weight-bearing activities, such as jogging, racquetball, tennis or high-impact aerobics. They might prefer low-impact exercises — low-impact aerobics, walking or stationary bicycling. Nonweight-bearing activities can be very effective for improving cardiovascular fitness, muscle strength and burning fat. They simply place less stress on joints and bones, reducing the possibility of injury.

To determine if the burner is on or off, simply remember that the more strenuous the activity, the greater number of calories burned. Even if you think the exercise is strenuous, if you are not exerting a high energy level, you won't burn as many calories as someone else performing the same activity for the same amount of time.

I recommend trying a variety of activities that don't require joining a health club. These might be exercises you can do in the privacy of your home while listening to music, or at work, walking about town over the noon hour or playing at the neighborhood recreational area. You don't have to stress your pocketbook. Whatever exercises you select, blend common sense, healthy balanced eating and some form of strength training or aerobic activity. Try to vary weekly routines to avoid boredom. You might want to try aerobic dance one day, swim the second and walk the third. Meet the experience as a challenge. Build your strength and endurance. It will be with you for many years to come. Exercising is effort well spent.

Select only those activities you enjoy most. Whatever you choose, make it something you could do for the rest of your life. You must make a firm commitment to exercise regularly — striving to be your fittest ever. Don't be defeated either if it takes you several months to work up enough endurance to do a 30-minute routine. Take it at your own pace.

The following list of activities with calories burned every 30 minutes of exercise, is based on the average metabolism of a 120-pound adult:

ACTIVITY	CALORIES BURNED/ 30 MINUTES
Aerobic Dancing	218
Bicycling	113
Calisthenics	120
Cross Country Skiing	325
General Housekeeping	115
Golf	170
Handball	225
Jogging	338
Racquetball	225
Squash	240
Swimming	173
Tennis	165
Walking Briskly	135
Weight Training	195
Yard Work	115

As an example, in order for an average 120-pound adult to "burn" off the calories in either a Taco Bellgrande Platter, an 8-inch Cousins Tuna Salad Submarine with potato chips and Coke or a Kentucky Fried Chicken "Extra Crispy" dinner, complete with mashed potato, gravy, coleslaw and roll, he or she would either have to walk 3 3/4 hours, swim 3 hours or go to an aerobic dance class for 2 1/4 hours. Choosing a Burger King Whopper, fries and a chocolate shake or McDonald's Quarter Pounder with cheese, fries and apple pie, would necessitate bicycling for 1 1/2 hours plus an hour each of swimming and jogging.

Checking Your Pulse

The best way you can determine if you are getting the maximum effect from exercise — enough to promote health and fitness yet not enough to overdo it — is to learn how to count your pulse rate and determine your maximum target heart zone. Most professionals recommend exercising at 70 to 75 percent of your maximum heart rate.

You can count your heartbeat over the left side of your chest, at your wrist on the thumb side, at the carotid artery just in front of the large vertical muscle felt in your neck next to your Adam's apple or at any convenient spot where you feel a pulse. To determine your 10-second and one-minute heart rate use the following formulas:

Resting pulse count X 10 = 10-second resting pulse count

10-second resting pulse count X 6 = one-minute resting heart rate

To find your resting pulse count while exercising it's necessary to find your pulse as quickly as possible immediately after stopping exercise and counting it for 10 seconds. Take that result and multiply it times 6 to find your one-minute resting heart rate.

Let's determine your target heart zone so you can compare it to your resting heart rate. The formula fo recalculating your target heart rate is as follows:

Take 220 minus your age times .75 divided by 6.

Here's an example for you to test these new formulas. What is a 32-year-old woman's target heart rate?

TARGET HEART RATE

Take 220	220
Minus Age 32	− 32
Equals	188
Multiply by .75 (75%)	x .75
Equals	141
Divide by 6	÷ 6
TARGET HEART RATE ZONE	23.5 rounded up to 24 beats in 10 seconds

24 X 6 = 144 beats per minute

10-second resting count X 6 = minute resting heart rate

The woman's target heart zone is 144 beats per minute or 24 heart beats per 10 seconds.

Exercising either below or above your target heart zone will not benefit your cardiovascular system. In fact, exercising to pulse rates above the zone can add a great deal of extra effort for very little improvement in fitness.

A delicate relationship exists between age, diet, behavior modification and exercise. After age 35, according to Dr. Rene Caillet and Leonard Gross's book *The Rejuvenation Strategy*, we need to be concerned with flexibility, lower-back strength and aerobic conditioning. You have to eat, think and feel right to perform healthful activities. Discipline yourself now so in years to come you can live life to the fullest.

Chapter 6

The Freezer in Your Fantasy

Frozen foods have become a staple in the American diet and fill one of the best sections of today's supermarkets.

If you have checked out the frozen food selection lately, you might find some surprises. In 1930, when commercial frozen foods were introduced, shoppers selected from a grand 27 items. Now we have some 1,500 to choose from. When Clarence Birdseye developed the first commercially feasible fast-freeze system in 1926, he could not have appreciated that he had only a bird's eye view of the present American pantry.

New frozen-food entrees have proliferated. In 1984 alone, 985 frozen food products were introduced, with 350 more in 1986. According to the National Frozen Food Association, retail sales of frozen foods totaled more than $18 billion in 1986. That sounds like a lot of cold cash, but consumers seem willing to spend this amount since the benefits far outweigh the higher cost of the product. Considering their freshness, nutrition, good taste, quality, convenience, no-waste and year-round availability, frozen foods offer incomparable value for the food dollar. Americans have never before had the diversity of quality, quantity and prices of frozen foods as they do in today's supermarkets.

Currently, the limited space in frozen food aisles is leading to wars among food manufacturers striving to develop the latest, greatest, tastiest food favorites. Some retailers have tried expanding their frozen food departments by 20 percent only to find they still don't have room to display all of the products available.

Frozen foods can and should be part of health and fitness regimens for the no-time-to-spare lifestyles of the 1990s. As mentioned earlier, Dr. Jean Mayer recently reported that there are "99 frozen dinners you can put on your shopping list." Of the 99, 44 dinners were highly recommended and met all of Mayer's nutri-

tional criteria.   The other 55 met all but one of his criteria.
Mayer's nutritional criteria consist of no more than 300 calories, a
maximum of 30 percent of calories from fat, no greater than 1,000
milligrams of sodium, and a minimum of one-third of the U.S.
RDAs for protein (15 grams) and a net weight of 9 ounces or
more.

Frozen foods can provide the variety, taste and fun often
sadly missing in "diet" programs.   And portion control, a common problem for dieters, isn't a problem.   Foods are packaged in
convenient single-serving, foil-cased tins or boil-in-bag pouches.
Manufacturers' cooking instructions permit flexibility too; most
foods can be heated in a conventional oven, toaster oven or
microwave.   Incidentally, the sales of frozen foods have soared as
microwave ovens have become more popular.   The combination
of frozen foods and microwaves is helping more and more folks
save energy, simplify clean-up and maintain unbeatable quality.
Almost 75 percent of American households have microwave
ovens. They're as standard as a toaster or coffee maker.

While frozen lunch and dinner staples have existed for years,
it's only in the last few years that breakfast entrees other than
egg substitutes, bagels and crumb cakes have been developed.
Sales of frozen breakfast food doubled from 1981 to 1986, and this
market is expected to hit $972 million in 1992.   One of the major
reasons this market is sure to expand is that today's adult often
eats only two meals — a hearty breakfast and a substantial supper.   Many of us can't get away at lunch because of our jobs.
Others choose to exercise rather than eat lunch.   Some people
skip lunch because it makes them feel tired.   Advertisers have
been quite successful in convincing us we must start our day
right with a "nutritious" breakfast.   Coffee and a donut just don't
make it whether you're an executive on Wall Street or a mother
on the go.

One no longer has to dine at McDonald's to enjoy a take-along
breakfast in the morning.   Swanson's has a terrific line of
Great Start microwaveable breakfast sandwiches and entrees.
In addition,   Sara Lee's elegant San Wich Croissants are filled
with   delectable   vegetables,   cheeses   and   various   breakfast
meats.   Even if caloric restrictions don't permit you to eat the
whole muffin, isn't half of something you love better than a
whole of something you don't like?   How about beginning your
day with a gooey cinnamon roll or Danish?   Believe it or not,
depending on the ingredients and nutritional make-up of these

foods, they might be all right. Look at the total fat, simple sugars and calories and see if these "fit" your needs. So why not let somebody else scramble the eggs, beat the batters and butter your toast? You can sleep a little later, exercise more, love yourself or mate, or do whatever else interests you besides cooking.

Lunch at work, home or on the go doesn't have to be the typical brown bag sandwich, cookies and fruit. Frozen french bread pizzas, egg rolls, spaghetti with meat balls, chili, Mexican foods or double-baked potatoes can be worked into your lunch buckets without guilt.

In addition to Stouffer's Lean Cuisine entrees, Weight Watchers and ConAgra's Light and Elegant meals are quality options. Other favorites include Armour's Classic Lite, the All American Gourmet Company's Slim Line, Campbell Soup's Le Menu line and Mrs. Paul's light fish entrees. Benihana and LaChoy have also taken a bite of the dinner action, introducing a line of frozen Oriental Lites and Fresh & Lite entrees. Offerings span everything from Italian chicken cacciatore to Oriental beef to the seafood-and-pasta lover's dream of linguini with scallops and clam sauce. Sound tempting? If these entrees sound too extravagant, how about southern fried chicken nuggets, lasagna or salisbury steak? And remember, chicken doesn't have to come from the Colonel to be "finger lickin' good." Tyson Foods' Chick 'N' Quick line of breaded breast fillets, patties or chunks are nutritious items that can easily be worked into your weight control plan. Mrs. Paul's, Booth's and Van De Kamp's lines of frozen fish dishes are almost sinfully good. Delectable sole fillets, salmon, cod, crab, shrimp and perch are but a few of the options available for light but satisfying meals. Sauced, breaded or served on a bed of rice or pasta, seafood offers a nice change for the beefeater. In addition, fattier fish such as salmon, whitefish, tuna and mackerel are rich in Omega-3 fatty acids. These acids appear to lower blood cholesterol and may reduce the risk of the nation's number one killer — coronary heart disease.

Does dessert always have to be limited to fruit? I should say not! Thanks to low-calorie, low-fat frozen desserts, sweet treats can be enjoyed daily for less than 200 calories. Who would ever believe that strawberry shortcake, German chocolate cake, cheesecake and heavenly chocolate mousse could be worked into a diet? Guiltless indulgences such as ice milk or soft-serve frozen yogurt cones also can be used on your weight loss program. A creamsicle or popsicle doesn't have to be a dreamed-sicle out of reach. Try savoring a lick of a sugar-free fudgsicle or any flavor of the original Popsicle. Nabisco Brands, makers of Lifesavers, the 9-calorie hard candy we've loved since childhood, recently introduced a frozen fruit pop in wild cherry, pineapple and orange that tastes terrific! And JELL-O Brand offers frozen gelatin and Pudding Pops, as well as natural fruit juice bars. If you prefer to satisfy your sweet cravings with fruit, check the label and buy the kinds without added sugar. You can select unsweetened frozen cherries, berries and mixed fruits year round. For fun, you can always top that frozen fruit, ice milk or yogurt with a dollop of non-dairy whipped topping.

What about frosty, frothy thirst quenchers? Sugar-free frozen beverages abound. Thirst-quenching, low-calorie lemonaid, fruit punch and orange drink are among the palate teasers ready to satisfy your desire for a sweet treat. Experiment by combining different flavors or adding club soda, Perrier or sugar-free tonic for a fizzy boost. Minute Maid's Light N' Juicy is an excellent drink that's worth trying. What have you got to lose for a measly 6 to 14 calories in a 6-ounce serving?

An evening at home can be as elegant as dining out at a fancy restaurant. Simply walk through the supermarket and select a meal to remember from the phenomenal array of frozen gourmet foods. Fantasies do come true. Light the candles, sit down, relax and enjoy convenience.

Chapter 7

Through the Arches — Your Way

Nutritionists, overzealous health advocates and governmental agencies have claimed "fast-food diets" increase a person's risk of nutritional deficiencies. Limited variety of foods is cited as the culprit. Lack of valuable nutrients, such as vitamins A, C and dietary fiber, are common. High fat, salt, sugar and calorie contents are risky. Processed foods, in particular, have been blamed for the increase in fat consumption over the past 75 years.

Are fast foods bad for us? Are the "junk foods" sure to lead to an early death? Fast-food franchises have been asked to print nutritional information on individual food wrappers, packages or pamphlets consumers can take home. While some chains have gathered this information, many have not. Unfortunately a federal law governing food labeling and ingredient listings doesn't exist for fast foods.

Officials at the National Restaurant Association aren't in favor of labeling fast foods. They believe consumers won't understand the chemical jargon on ingredient lists. Moreover, recipes and ingredients change constantly, making it impractical and costly to label items. Since consumers often favor taste over nutrition, many restaurants claim labeling would be useless. It's "after-the-fact information." Consumers have already purchased the product so what's the use of telling them what is in it?

The National Restaurant Association's solution to this dilemma is to encourage consumers to ask for information. Still, how can we expect good answers when no one has researched the questions? Furthermore, many managers at fast-food chains are uninformed and can't answer nutrition questions. They generally tell customers to write to their corporate headquarters.

Why is there a lack of information about fast foods? First, most products haven't been analyzed. There's no information, good or bad, to report. Second, chains don't want to release "trade secret" ingredients. Third, development of nutrition guides, advertisements and education campaigns would be very costly. Finally, advertisers bent on promoting fun and fast times with burgers, fries and chocolate malts probably would be restricted.

Unfortunately, it's often difficult for consumers to evaluate fast foods. Advertising often is misleading. Some chains say their food is "healthy," but their definitions of healthy face stiff opposition in the medical community.

I agree with food critics and health specialists who want fast foods labeled and ads spelling out ingredients. Presenting a product in its best possible light may be business smart but nutritionally dumb. Such selectivity could backfire. In fact, selective advertising may work against restaurants that have jumped on the nutrition-advertising bandwagon. Instead of warding off labeling legislation, selective ads are more likely to encourage government to push even harder for ingredient breakdowns on packages.

Marketers should promote the positive nutritional advantages of their products over their competitors'. Think about it — advertisers do it with cereal, peanut butter and ice cream, so why not with fast foods? Show us comparisons of an "original" version compared with a newly formulated lower calorie, sodium and fat choice.

Nutritional analysis could include calories, protein, carbohydrates, fat, cholesterol, sodium and percentages of the recommended allowances for essential vitamins and minerals. In turn, marketing should cover all these nutritional factors, permitting us to key in to our nutritional interests and needs. Nutritional information could be displayed in magazine advertisements, newspapers or even at carry-out windows.

Many of you might think nutritional information wouldn't influence the one-third of the 66 million Americans eating out every day. If, in fact, it influenced only 1 percent of this group, that would mean 220,000 people would be affected. Isn't it well worth the effort?

While consumers haven't cut back on fast foods, health is a major reason they're not eating more of it. If we could enjoy fast food "our way," would we be able to make a "balanced meal" out of it? Can the "original" great taste of fast food stand up to a nutritional change for the better? Are consumers sauced, dipped and fried out — ready to expand taste centers and sample food in its unblanketed bare "naturalness?"

Consumers do care about their eating habits and are health conscious. We are making more prudent food selections — both at home and away. According to a 1983 Gallup survey, six out of every ten consumers eat more fruits, vegetables and whole grains than in the past. In addition, many of us have tried to cut back on refined sugars, animal fats and salt. Because concerned consumers express interest in healthier fast foods, restaurants have changed their menus. The result is more salad bars, fresh fruits, leaner cuts of meat and poultry and fresh seafood. Some restaurants now use less filler and additives and have switched from animal to vegetable fats for frying. Look at the number of "heart-healthy" menu selections restaurants offer. Fast-food chains could improve their images by doing the same.

All fast foods aren't "junk." However, any food, fast or otherwise, should be eaten in moderation, providing the consumer is healthy and free of dietary restrictions. A total fast-food diet or use of foods containing lots of sugar, fat or "empty calories" is not recommended. Still, some fast-food choices can be healthy. Easy, simple food quickly prepared with a minimum of fat, salt and calories can be healthy, particularly if you cut the fat and add fiber.

Most people don't want to be limited to eating burgers, fries, pizza and submarine sandwiches. Everyone needs a variety of foods. Dieters in particular seem to crave fattening fast foods. They feel deprived, especially if they like hanging out at the "Happy Days" spots. When this happens, it's better to have a couple slices of cheese pizza rather than make pizza totally off limits. You're more likely to wolf down a whole pepperoni pizza with extra cheese if you can't have any. Many consumers don't know that some fast foods, such as cheese pizza with vegetable toppings, is good food, providing nutrients from all essential food groups. Portion control is the key.

We shouldn't expect people to live in a vacuum or go "cold turkey." Despite the hundreds of diet books, spas and fitness clubs, "yo-yo" dieting continues because of a disregard for realistic expectations. If a diet looks good on paper, but tastes like cardboard, how long do you guess someone will stick with it? If you have to spend hours planning menus, purchasing special foods, preparing and cleaning up, it stands to reason that programs will be abandoned.

We know from research studies that our behavior influences our health. We also know that preventive nutritional guidelines can and do influence our health — not only for today, but for the rest of our lives. Healthy diets and fitness must become a way of life. But, it's unrealistic to assume that people will just learn to do without. To believe you simply won't eat any more potato chips, chocolate chip cookies, ice cream or spare ribs is not realistic. Trade-offs are the name of the game.

Having it your way is easier than you think if you understand these four fast food facts:

1. All fast foods are not bad for us.

2. It's not enough to hold the pickle, relishes and sauces.

3. You aren't always making a healthier choice when you select fish or chicken instead of beef.

4. Selecting a salad isn't always a wise decision for dieters.

A single broiled hamburger or junior roast beef sandwich has roughly half the calories (225-250) of a fried fillet of fish or chicken sandwich with 435 or 510 calories, respectively. Fish and chicken are only best when baked or broiled without added fat. Salads dressed with regular creamy-style or oil-based dressing, mayonnaise, cheese, bacon bits, olives, nuts, seeds, pickle chips or croutons are high in fat, calories and sodium. You can add an extra 1,000 calories and more than a day's allowance for sodium by using a quarter cup of regular salad dressing, 2 ounces of cheese, bacon bits, a handfull of nuts and a few olives.

The trick is finding a salad bar with lots of plain undressed fresh vegetables and fruit fixings. Stack your plate with piles of greens, cauliflower, broccoli, carrots, cucumber and peppers. They are low in calories, filling and high in fiber.

It's best to select fresh fruits rather than canned or mixed fruits containing added sugar. Dress your salads with low-calorie stretchers that don't contain a lot of sodium, such as lemon juice, flavored vinegars, low-sodium tomato or vegetable juice and mixtures of freshly ground herbs. While low-calorie salad dressings contain relatively few calories, they are often high in sodium. So use them sparingly.

Go easy on high-protein and fat ingredients, too, such as peas and beans, cheese and assorted diced meats or fish. If it's easier for you to diet with prepackaged foods instead of serving yourself, try McDonald's line of ready-made salads including Chef, Shrimp and Garden Vegetable. Hardees, Wendy's and Burger King also have complete salad bar services. And next time, try enjoying a cup of soup, chili or a plain baked potato with your salad, instead of the typical burger and fries.

A more detailed discussion of the Do's and Don'ts with fast foods is found in Chapter Four. However, generally speaking, it's best to avoid French fried, breaded or sauced fast-food fare. Foods prepared in saturated fats — potatoes made in lard or coconut oil or eggs fried in butter — should also be avoided by the heart smart and calorie wise. In addition, steer clear of high-fat, high-cholesterol sausages, bacon or muffin-type sandwiches containing these ingredients.

Limit selections high in simple sugars, malted milks, sundaes and hot apple pies. The simpler the better! In other words, stick to single or junior versions of grilled sandwiches instead of a double- or triple-decker delight. Skip the cheese, layers of bacon, sauces and condiments. And whenever possible, select or take along fresh fruit, plain vegetables and whole-grain bread.

You can make trade-offs. If you eat something high in fat and calories at one meal, limit fats the rest of the day. *The Expresslane Diet's* Exchange System for fast foods shows you how to substitute or trade staples for an occasional fast-food indulgence.

The name of the game for consumers is to make their food preferences known to fast-food franchises. To win the wrestling match with restauranteurs and chain managers, you need only follow this three-step process: First and foremost, make your food preferences known. Next, request complete ingredient and nutritional information from all food chains. And finally, make sure your requests have been met by local as well as national fast-food franchises. You can have it your way!

Chapter 8

Consumer Power: Make Your Voice Heard

According to the *39th Annual Consumer Expenditures Study (CES)* published in September 1986, total grocery store sales in 1985 rose 4.7 percent above the preceding year. Weekly spending approximated $58.85 per household or $21.43 per person. But how are Americans doling out these food dollars?

The Food Book, a 1985 guide to the most popular brand-name foods in the U.S., says that Americans spent more than $190 billion or 60 percent of every food dollar on brand-name convenience foods. The *Supermarket Business* journal emphasizes that shoppers' interest in frozen foods, in particular, is hot and should continue to "heat up."

In the mid-1980s, Americans spent about $3.6 billion each year for frozen convenience and prepared foods, with frozen dinners leading the pack. Nearly $1.6 billion went for "TV" dinners alone. Sales of other prepared products such as pizza, Oriental dinners and meat-filled pies also blossomed, exhibiting substantial outlays of $1.7 billion, $213 million and $227 million, respectively, in 1985. On other food fronts, because of increased availability of refrigerated and shelf-stable fruit juices, frozen concentrated fruit juice sales dropped 0.62 percent. However, frozen fruit drinks showed a gain of 5.2 percent in 1985, representing $135 million in sales. And to think I thought the flattened purchase curve for fruit juices meant people were more concerned about getting more fiber from fresh fruits.

What about fresh-frozen vegetables? Produce departments in grocery stores have seen radical transformation. In fact, canned food companies have already begun to enter the fresh produce market. Avocados, kiwi, mango, Oriental vegetables and the like have gone from upscale oddities to staples. In the past ten years, supermarkets have progressed from providing an average of 85 produce items to an average of 250 items. According to the National American Wholesaler-Grocers' Association, produce departments are becoming "huge gardens" that may carry as many as 400 items. If produce departments continue to tout vegetables that are ready pared, peeled, bunched, diced or sliced, their popularity is certain to climb. This represents a healthy addition to menus using convenience foods. We are witnessing a definite change in American lifestyles and food patterns. Today, fresh produce is the first choice for many consumers. Freshfrozen fruits and vegetables are a close second and their canned counterparts are a distant third. Nonetheless, all foods have a place if well planned.

Manufacturers continue to offer new or reformulated products in the hopes of maintaining a spot in the frozen-food section and consumer's cart. Some might even call this ploy "frozen Darwinism."

The freezer case can serve consumers around the clock, whether it's a traditional bagel on the run, micro burgers and soup or an elegant gourmet dinner followed by an exotic frozen dessert. Many of the items are specially prepared and calorie-reduced — perfect for dieters.

What about the purchases of frozen "diet foods?" It's not easy to categorize "diet foods," to understand the differences between lite, calorie-reduced or dietetic foods, or to quantify the amount of money we spend on them. This is because so many different products are available, with many overlaps into "other" food categories. Statistical information is scant at best. Bearing that in mind, experts have estimated that in 1986, frozen prepared "diet foods" accounted for approximately one-third of the frozen merchandise and 40 percent of the gross sales of $3.7 billion. Skeptics might think manufacturers preserve their shares in the competitive frozen food market by creating a "diet" or "light" version of their products.

Some consumers associate negatives — high cost or less taste — with foods for special diet plans. Part of the marketing problem rests in unique individual perceptions. For instance, some people think of yogurt as a low-fat, low-calorie nutritious food because advertisers have promoted that concept. In fact, some yogurts are prepared with whole-milk solids and sugar-sweetened fruit. They contain a lot more calories than plain low-fat yogurt, not to mention less calcium.

Consumers should recognize that "diet foods" aren't neces-sarily low in calories, fat or sodium. Very often, the proportion of key nutrients, such as fats, are high, while other valuable nutri-ents, such as carbohydrates, are sacrificed. Some packaged mixes, soups, condiments and canned goods may be low in fats and calories, but very high in sodium. And the same applies to "lite" foods — lower calories but high sodium. Then too, even low-fat foods are risky if the fat that is there is "saturated," which raises cholesterol. Word and mind games rule. Shoppers play them in rationalizing purchases, and food producers play them to win a buck.

It's not enough that we purchase brand-name nutrition guides and become active label readers. We have to learn which nutrients are key, how much is too much, how to translate these values into daily nutrient requirements and how best to combine food selections to ensure nutritional adequacy.

Food guides such as *The Food Book: A Complete Guide to the Most-Popular Names in the United States,* by Bert Stern, Lawrence Chilnick and Lynn Sonberg; Barbara Kraus's *Complete Guide to Sodium,* as well as her other guides on calories and car-bohydrates; Pennington and Church's *Food Values of Portions Commonly Used*; Jean Carper's *The Brand-Name Nutrition Counter*; and Dr. Michael Jacobson's *Fast-Food Guide* are a few of the resources marketed to help bridge the nutrition informa-tion gap. These guides partially meet consumers' needs. They afford an opportunity to compare brand-name, convenience, pro-cessed, fast and "natural" foods. The typical food profile includes ingredients, portions, calories, protein, carbohydrates, fat, sodium, cholesterol, fiber and the U.S. RDA for vitamins and minerals. Some also include grams of saturated versus unsatu-rated fat and total grams of simple versus complex sugars (carbo-hydrates). Dr. Michael Jacobson's book, *The Fast-Food Guide,* even gives readers a "gloom rating" system to apply when eating out at a fast-food spot.

Teaching consumers what's in their food and how to select the best products at the supermarket or restaurant is good. However, the average consumer doesn't have the time nor inter-est to decipher the data. It's not enough to give consumers prudent dietary guidelines: restrict sodium to between 1,100 to 3,300 milligrams per day; eat between 50 and 60 percent of calories as carbohydrates with emphasis on complex carbohydrates; increase dietary fiber to 20 to 30 grams per day; limit total fat consumption to no more than 30 percent of total daily calories. What do these numbers mean to the average person? How do you calculate these things? How do you put this information together to attain and maintain a lean, healthy physique, busy lifestyle and still enjoy living? This is not easy for the convenience eater — which is the real issue at hand.

The bottom line rests with total daily dietary composition — not one or two values of selected foods. *The Expresslane Diet* lets you see the entire nutritional picture without playing games or having to make tedious computations. All the calculations have been done for you.

As the saying goes, everything is in a name. The fact the name "Weight Watchers" may trigger negative emotions in some people explains why advertisers have focused on the great taste of their products rather than on the name. Whatever the game, consumers still hold the trump card in the supermarket. We have the choice of buying or denying food purchases. You can be in the winner's circle.

Chapter 9

What Lies Ahead?

By the year 2000, more than 50 percent of all food dollars will be spent in restaurants. Microwave ovens will be in 90 percent of American households, so most foods will be microwaveable. Food shoppers will be purchasing simple finger, one-handed commuter and portable foods. More foods will be shelf-stable and refrigerator alternatives. Emphasis will be on low-calorie snacks to please grazing appetites and desires to remain slim. Then, too, we'll be consuming more frozen, premium quality, light entrees and toasting our meals with champagne. It will be an era of simple elegance.

Amidst all the talk about increased consumption of prepared, take-out and fast foods, there are some experts who disagree. Faith Popper, chairwoman and chief executive officer of Brain Reserve, a New York research firm, predicts Americans will turn away from fast foods and return to many of the 1950s trends and lifestyle. Entrepreneurial women will run businesses in their homes. Home-cooked meals will become fashionable. Families will reunite. Outside entertainment will be the exception to the rule. All of these changes will occur as a direct result of the cocooning craze that's already under way in American homes today.

Still, life stresses and work pressures will continue to promote a need for relief from decision making. Instead of seeking fun outside the home, families will stay home and entertain themselves. They will enjoy the comforts of lounging in relaxed furniture, pushing buttons to turn on VCRs, television sets and stereos and maybe even taking part in good conversation and great food.

Baby making is going to come back, too. Futurists perceive the typical couple as having two, three or even four kids, as opposed to the 1980s DINKS (Dual Income, No Kids) or YUPPIE couples with approximately 1.8 children.

While Americans will prepare more home-cooked meals, they will do so with less work. That means they'll be relying on many more convenience-type products — fresh, frozen, ready-made or shelf-stable.

A new consumer movement similar to the Ralph Nader era is also scheduled to show up in the '2000s. Fortunately, this movement is supposed to be pro-health. People will speak up and reject foods they know to be unhealthy. Consumers will think nothing of calling ahead to restaurants — even fast-food restaurants — to request specially broiled meats, oven-browned or baked starches and steamed plain fresh vegetables as opposed to fried, buttered or breaded alternatives. And like today, chains will be welcome options. Supposedly national toll-free telephone numbers will be available so customers can register complaints, make recommendations, request nutritional information or ask any questions regarding fast foods 24 hours of any day. Customers will also have the option of charging fast food to credit cards.

Even though patterns of food consumption fluctuate like clothing styles, American diets will always have a place for fruits, vegetables and grains. This is apparent in the latest 30-year retrospective food consumption findings from the U.S. Department of Agriculture's economic research group. They predict Americans will continue to eat more poultry, fish and other lean meat substitutes, such as trimmed pork and veal. Use of fattier cuts of beef and lamb will continue to decline. Skim milk and low-fat dairy product consumption should increase, compared with whole milk or high-fat products. Healthful salad bars will become ubiquitous. Supermarkets and restaurants will have fresh fruit and vegetable bonanzas. Sauces, dressings and toppings will contain polyunsaturated and monounsaturated fats and oils since Americans will continue to avoid lard, butter and other saturated fats. Sales of foods containing refined sugars will plummet as natural fruit juices or fresh fruits reign supreme. We won't be wetting our whistles with much hard liquor or beer either. Unfortunately, we will probably continue to prefer soft drinks over milk, juice and other beverages.

Won't Americans continue to enjoy life in the fast-food lane? Will social trends really take us revisiting the '50s in the '2000s? Whether you're discussing future American cuisine, dining styles, shopping patterns or health, one thing is certain: Lifestyles of today will dictate standards of tomorrow. Americans are not the fickle buying public they are sometimes made out to be.

To speculate on what and how Americans will be eating post year 2000, let's examine some futuristic models of tomorrow's consumers, supermarkets and restaurants. Most experts agree: Fast foods and convenience dining are here to stay!

Mr. Spock would have future shock were he to visit a supermarket in the 21st Century. Tomorrow's customers undoubtedly will enjoy "one-stop shopping" amidst sleekly styled supermarket warehouses, providing a vast array of simple and fancy ready-made meals. The only downside could be the customer-operated checkerless scanners used at check-out.

At the supermarket industry's 50th anniversary convention in 1987, futurists and industry analysts posed three very different models for tomorrow's supermarkets. The first model included a huge multi-level modular complex resembling today's shopping mall. It featured a wide variety of food and non-food items. Consumers would be able to park on the rooftop, taking elevators down to shop on separate levels for perishables and non-perishable groceries. Complexes would include take-out, fast-food delivery services and child-care companions. For relaxation, private lounge areas would be located in beautifully decorated alcoves. Modular expansions would permit greater flexibility, too. Expansions, revisions or deletions could be as easy as plugging in additional units, including customer operated check-out systems for fast in-and-out self service, or adding convenience store sections having their own separate entrances, exits and check-outs. Complexes would be open 24 hours a day.

The second model uses a computer-generated order system. Customers would have phone-in delivery service. Their orders would be delivered directly to their homes. Home delivery service wouldn't be limited to food staples either. All you'll need is extra money for delivery charges. Car phones will become the standard so customers can phone on the way home and have ready-made foods waiting when they reach the front door. As for shoppers who would rather see what they're buying, they still could choose to drive to the supermarket warehouses. Goods could be selected from video displays and picked up at a nearby dispensing station. Shopping carts would be a thing of the past. Instead, shoppers would use electronic wands or cards. They would walk up and down aisles, select from permanent displays and pick up bagged orders on their way out of the store. This model could run on very low overhead.

The third supermarket model, my personal favorite, is very theatrical. People would shop in a series of fancy, dramatically lit stages where in-house chefs would present cooking demonstrations and prepare nutritious and fun meals before your eyes. Menus would include top-quality fresh foods and gourmet lines of frozen or ready-prepared products available in the store. One of the goals in this system would be to encourage people to either purchase ingredients to make these dishes themselves, or to buy the prepared products directly from the chef's in-store kitchen. Home delivery service, fast foods, catering, cooking and nutrition classes would be offered under this supermarket umbrella. This model is one-stop shopping with a flair!

Contrary to Ms. Popcorn's projections, Mona Doyle, food industry consultant, believes that "ready-to-eat" foods will become as important as ready-to-wear clothing. Other analysts voice similar views, projecting that by the year 2000 as much or possibly more cooking will be done in supermarkets as in homes.

The food industry is going to have to ready itself for an older, more affluent buying public as well. Since more than one-quarter of the American population will be over 65 by 1990, there will be an influx of older, more affluent shoppers who will be demanding convenience products of good quality.

Selection and display of products in supermarkets will not be left to chance either. Even though shelf space is limited, given more floor space and advanced technology, layouts will be more flexible and able to handle many more new products. They will need to be. In the first six months of 1987 alone, 4,865 new food items were introduced to supermarkets. This is 20 percent higher than the number of products introduced for that same period in 1986. The number of new products entering the market by 2000, by some estimates, approximates an increase of 280 percent.

Future stores will devote a tremendous amount of space to areas for microwave ovens. Supermarket shoppers will be able to pick out a frozen or fresh ready-made convenience item and pop it into the microwave while shopping. This eat-it-and-run feature will promote competition between supermarkets and fast-food chains. Location and delivery service options could well be the principle factors in the competition equation.

Supermarket shelves in the year 2000 probably won't contain many low-cost generic items. These products are already declining in supermarkets today. Quality above all, even if the price is higher, will take priority. Customers will take advantage of new product lines and food products. Supermarket departments will be re-scaled to include full-service delis with built-in catering services, health, beauty and pharmaceutical departments, bakeries and larger staple areas for produce, frozen foods, poultry, meat and fish.

What's happening to restaurants? Today's lifestyle trends indicate that the buzz words for tomorrow's restaurant include fast, convenient and hassle-free. However, they will be fast in a much different sense of the word than we think of it today. Customers will be enjoying more healthful, old-fashioned fast-food flavors. The days of trendy, unhealthy fast foods will disappear. They will be replaced by fast foods that will taste great and be good for you, too.

Diners will continue to want convenience. While today 50 percent of American women traditionally responsible for home-cooked meals are working outside the home, by the end of this century, the figure is expected to climb to about 75 percent. In the future, workers will have more options for healthy lunches. Futurist Jerome C. Glenn, with the Washington D.C.-based Partnership for Productivity International, predicts the entrance of electronic food delivery services. Food will be carted throughout downtown areas to service tens of thousands of workers. Other futurists foresee package innovations that will give a whole new meaning to the carry-out business. Mail meals, freeze-dried and irradiated food innovations will be common. These packaging ideas will fit well with the needs of our aging population.

Two wage-earner households, better able to afford the top-quality convenience, will mean more variety on the market. Families won't be satisfied existing on convenience microwaveable munchies alone. Many foods considered more or less exotic today, such as wild mushrooms, star fruit or leechie nuts, will be common purchases.

What the restaurant of the 21st Century will look like remains unknown. Futurists submit only two kinds of restaurants will survive — fast-food and fine-dining establishments. Within the next 20 years, the restaurant industry could be hit by a wave of totally machine-staffed cafes. Servers of the future could well be programed robots that deliver food to tables, joke or play games with kids and sing tunes from the Top 40. Looking on the brighter side, robot characters, unlike people, will only need an occasional day off, don't demand tips and won't be disagreeable or sassy to customers. A 4-foot tall, 180-pound robot server named TANBO R-1 has already been introduced in Pasadena, California, at the "Two Panda Robot" restaurant.

In many restaurants, patrons will merely feed credit cards into table side slots or touch screens to place food orders and trigger pickups. The gold card craze remains and moves to fast-food restaurants as well. When dining at a fast-food spot, you'll simply place your order and watch robot chefs put everything together.

In lieu of this push-button elegance, there will also be a renewed appreciation for fine personalized dining service. Some people will want to be waited on and pampered by real people, not robots. They will, however, find it somewhat disconcerting to learn that robots will be preparing their foods anyway. The personal service provided by real people will be much more expensive. In fact, for the first time, servers are going to be in the driver's seat of the food industry. The Labor Department estimates that by 1995, the need for servers will increase by more than 30 percent. Serving will not only become more lucrative, but also much easier. Loads will be lightened by ergonomically designed shoes and high-tech, low-weight cookware and dinnerware. As customers will be electronically ordering foods, servers will be freed of tasks such as taking food orders and running back and forth between tables. Food orders will be electronically transmitted by servers to robots in the kitchen using portable computer pads.

The Expresslane Diet has come at a momentous time. The time is ripe for dissemination and understanding of good nutrition information on fast and convenience food. The coming years should bring many more wholesome fast-food choices for consumers. This will take place because we will express our needs for wholesome convenience.

The Expresslane Diet will help you become a wiser convenience shopper. Take your pick — convenience at the supermarket, fast-food chain, micromagic machine or any other quick-fix spot. And even if you're one of the few who will be doing the cooking, I'd bet you'll still be looking in the Yellow Pages for helping hands or scouting a quick, nutritious bite every now and then.